D0515498

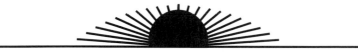

GREAT MINDS OF SCIENCE

Jonas Salk

Creator of the Polio Vaccine

Salvatore Tocci

Enslow Publishers, Inc.

40 Industrial Road   PO Box 38
Box 398   Aldershot
Berkeley Heights, NJ 07922 Hants GU12 6BP
USA   UK

http://www.enslow.com

Copyright © 2003 by Salvatore Tocci.

All rights reserved.

No part of this book may be reproduced by any means
without the written permission of the publisher.

Library of Congress Cataloging-in-Publication Data

Tocci, Salvatore.
  Jonas Salk : creator of the polio vaccine / Salvatore Tocci.
     p. cm. — (Great minds of science)
Summary: A biography of the American doctor and medical researcher who
helped to develop successful influenza and polio vaccines, then turned
his attention to vaccines for cancer and AIDS prevention.
Includes bibliographical references and index.
  ISBN 0-7660-2097-5
  1. Salk, Jonas, 1914—-Juvenile literature. 2. Virologists—United
States—Biography—Juvenile literature. 3. Poliomyelitis
vaccine—Juvenile literature. [1. Salk, Jonas, 1914– 2. Scientists. 3.
Poliomyelitis vaccine.] I. Title. II. Series.
QR31.S25 T63 2002
610'.92—dc21

                            2002003888

Printed in the United States of America

10 9 8 7 6 5 4 3 2 1

To Our Readers:
We have done our best to make sure all Internet addresses in this book were
active and appropriate when we went to press. However, the author and the
publisher have no control over and assume no liability for the material
available on those Internet sites or on other Web sites they may link to. Any
comments or suggestions can be sent by e-mail to comments@enslow.com or
to the address on the back cover.

Illustration Credits: Courtesy of the family of Jonas Salk and the
Jonas Salk Trust, pp. 22, 24, 41; Courtesy of the Salk Institute for
Biological Studies, pp. 103, 107; Franklin D. Roosevelt Library,
pp. 28, 92; Library of Congress, pp. 34, 57; March of Dimes, pp. 16,
37, 48, 52, 54, 64, 66, 69, 72, 78, 86, 89, 99,; National Library of
Medicine, pp. 9, 75; National Library of Medicine, Hal Rumel, p. 13.

Cover Illustration: © Dennis Kunkel Microscopy, Inc. (background);
AP/Wide World Photos (inset).

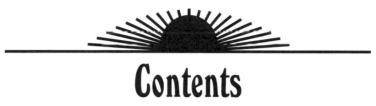

Contents

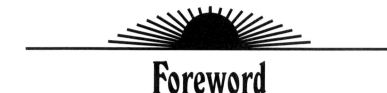

Foreword

The development of the killed poliovirus vaccine was a pivotal event in the mid-twentieth century, both scientifically and socially. Within six years, it brought under control in the United States a disease that was the frightening epidemic of its time— a disease even more frightening for most people than AIDS is today. It was the first practical use of techniques that permitted viruses to be grown in bottles. The nationwide field trial run by Dr. Thomas Francis in 1954 was the largest ever conducted and set the standard for controlled field trials of vaccines. New methods had to be developed by the U.S. government for approval and monitoring of the killed poliovirus vaccine, methods that continue to influence the FDA today.

It was the first demonstration that a viral disease could be controlled successfully with a vaccine made from noninfectious (dead) viruses. Since the time of Pasteur it had been believed that only infectious (live) viruses would work in vaccines. A live virus vaccine was later developed for polio that could be given orally (by mouth), but it occasionally caused polio in people who received it or others who came in contact with them. The injected killed poliovirus vaccine cannot cause polio. The U.S. Public Health Service now recommends that only the killed poliovirus vaccine be used in the United States.

The fight against polio was supported by the largest private fund-raising effort ever: The March of Dimes. There was very little government or industry support for vaccine development at the time. The polio vaccine truly belonged to the people of this country—they paid for it themselves with millions and millions of nickels and dimes and dollars and with countless hours of volunteer effort.

It is easy to look back now and make these kinds of summary statements. But what is part of history for students today were everyday events for me and my friends. Salvatore Tocci has done a commendable job, writing an accurate account that brings the details of these events within the grasp of young people of the twenty-first century. What makes history exciting for students is realizing that it is the story of people just like themselves.

Darrell Salk, M.D.
September 12, 2002

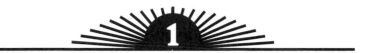

Innocent Victims

FROM THE 1930s INTO THE EARLY 1950s, parents all across America were afraid that their child might be the next victim. What parents feared was a disease called polio. They knew that a child who got polio could become paralyzed for life. A child could even die from the disease. Parents were especially afraid because polio was spreading rapidly throughout America and no one knew why.

Some people thought that flies or fleas were responsible for spreading polio. Others believed that the disease was caught by eating contaminated fruit. Still others felt that someone could get polio by swimming in contaminated water.

However it spread, polio was more likely to strike a child than an adult.

To protect their children, some parents tied pieces of cloth soaked in camphor around their child's neck. They believed that this strong-smelling chemical would keep their child safe from polio. If they could, parents who lived in cities sent their children to the countryside during the summer. A child was more likely to get polio in warmer weather, especially in a crowded city. Those families who remained in the cities often did not allow their children to go swimming or play with friends. Many people stayed at home as much as possible.

A doctor working in a Minneapolis hospital in the late 1940s reported that the "people in Minneapolis were so frightened that there was nobody in the restaurants. There was practically no traffic, the stores were empty. It was considered a feat of [bravery] almost to go out and mingle in public." The doctor pointed out that people had good reason to be afraid. "We admitted 464 proven cases of polio just at the University Hospital, which is unbelievable. . . . Maybe two or

QUARANTINE
POLIOMYELITIS

All persons are forbidden to enter or leave these premises without the permission of the HEALTH OFFICER under PENALTY OF THE LAW.

    This notice is posted in compliance with the SANITARY CODE OF CONNECTICUT and must not be removed without permission of the HEALTH OFFICER.

Form D-1-Po.   _____Health Officer.

A quarantine notice was sometimes used in cases of polio. The practice of quarantining (isolating patients) was not very effective in preventing polio, however, because the disease was often spread by people with mild cases who were not even aware they were ill.

three hours after a lot of these kids would come in with a stiff neck or a fever, they'd be dead. It was unbelievable."[1]

Despite the precautions parents took, polio quickly became an epidemic in America. (An epidemic is a disease that spreads rapidly over a large geographic area. As a result, many people become infected in just a short time.) In 1940, about 10,000 cases of polio were reported in America. In 1949, the number of people who got polio skyrocketed to more than 42,000.[2] One of those victims was a twelve-year-old girl named Peg Schulze, a seventh-grade student who lived in Austin, Minnesota.

One day in September of 1949, Peg was in chorus class, but her mind was on the home-coming parade scheduled for that afternoon. For the past week, she and her friends had spent all their spare time working on their class float. They were sure it would win the award for first place. As Peg sang in class, she suddenly felt the muscles in her left leg twitch. The muscles twitched so violently that they made her skirt pop up and down against her leg.

Peg tried to calm the muscles by pressing hard on her leg. But they still kept twitching violently. She tried to tighten the muscles by extending her leg. She also stretched her leg forward and rotated her ankle. Nothing worked. When chorus class was over, she headed for her locker. As Peg was walking in the hall, her legs buckled, and she fell to the ground. A classmate thought she had fainted. She helped Peg get back on her feet. Feeling a little better, Peg walked home for lunch as she usually did every day.

Two days earlier, she had had a sore throat and a mild headache. Afraid that her mother would keep her home, Peg said nothing about what had happened in school. She did not want to miss the homecoming activities that afternoon. Besides, Peg felt that she would feel better if she had something to eat. But when she reached for a glass of milk, her hand started to shake. She tried holding the glass with both hands. Her hands shook so much that the milk spilled out of the glass. Now there was no way to hide that something was wrong from her mother.

Peg's mother felt the girl's forehead. When she sensed that it was hot, she told Peg to go right to bed and went to call the doctor. He came right away and took Peg's temperature. He found that she had a high fever. When the doctor returned the next morning, he told Peg's parents to take her to the hospital where he could check her more closely. Just one day after she was happily singing and thinking about homecoming, Peg was told she had polio. She remembered the doctor telling her: "You will need to go to a special hospital for polio patients, in Minneapolis."[3] The next day, Peg found herself paralyzed from the neck down.

Despite what most people believed at that time, only about one percent of those who got polio became paralyzed. Most of its victims suffered only a sore throat, headache, and diarrhea. In fact, someone who became infected with polio might never develop any symptoms at all. But polio was spreading rapidly and infecting many people, especially those living in cities. Even though only one percent became paralyzed because of polio, this was still a large number of people. If polio continued to spread, then more and more innocent victims would become paralyzed. Many more would also die.

Doctors could offer little help in stopping the spread of polio. For one thing, they had nothing to treat those who caught the disease. All they could do was to suggest that those who became paralyzed, like Peg, go to a special hospital. Here

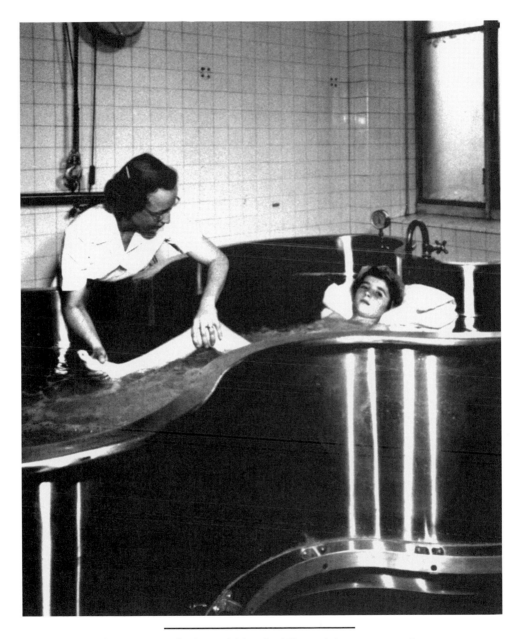

A polio patient soaks in a whirlpool while receiving treatment from a physical therapist in 1949.

nurses applied hot packs to try to relax their muscles. Paralyzed patients were also given special exercises to stretch their muscles. But the patients hated the treatments. As Peg put it, "I was sure my skin was being blistered and burned [from the hot packs]."[4] As for the exercises, "[they] hurt all the time."[5]

One thing that doctors did know was what caused polio. It was a virus. A virus is an extremely small particle that can cause disease. The only way to see a virus is with the help of a very powerful microscope. Viruses are not considered living things. To make more viruses, they must infect a living cell.

Once it has infected a cell, the virus takes control. It turns the infected cell into a virus factory. Hundreds of new viruses are made inside the cell. Eventually, these viruses break open the cell, killing it. All these viruses then search for more cells to infect. This process continues, unless it is somehow stopped. Unfortunately, doctors had no way to stop the poliovirus.

The poliovirus was first identified in 1908 by

two doctors in Austria. The next year, hospitals started recording cases of polio in America. The first epidemic of polio occurred in 1916. Over 9,000 cases were reported just in New York City that year.[6]

Today, doctors realize that there are actually three different polioviruses, called types I, II, and III. All three types can enter the body through the mouth and nose. The poliovirus enters when a person drinks contaminated water, comes in contact with a surface where the virus is present, or is exposed to droplets from the cough or sneeze of an infected person. After entering the mouth, the virus passes through the throat and stomach and then enters the intestines. The virus infects cells in both the throat and intestines, making many more new viruses. In most people, these viruses cause no more than the symptoms of a cold or a case of diarrhea. The viruses then pass out the body, leaving the person unharmed.

In some people, however, the viruses pass from the intestines into the bloodstream. Streaming through the blood, the viruses reach

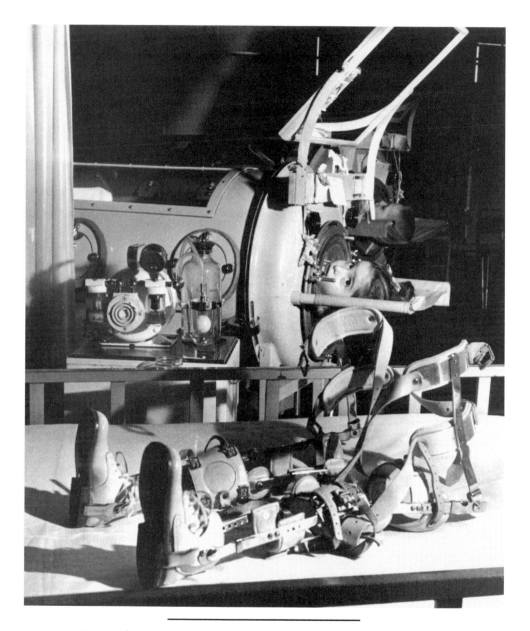

Some polio patients required iron lungs to aid them in breathing. Iron lungs enclosed the entire body except the head. Others needed metal braces for their legs in order to stand or walk.

nerves that control the muscles of the legs, arms, and abdomen. If the viruses attack and kill these nerves, then these muscles become paralyzed. The more nerve cells destroyed, the greater the paralysis. The poliovirus can also reach the base of the brain. If these brain cells are destroyed, then the muscles that control swallowing become paralyzed. Muscles that control the movement of the eyes, tongue, face, and neck also become paralyzed. This is the most serious form of polio. This is the type of polio that Peg developed in 1949.

Fortunately for Peg, her condition improved. About five months after she had entered the polio hospital, Peg went home. She could now walk a few steps by herself. She could walk even farther with the help of her crutches, or "walking sticks," as she called them. Two months later, Peg returned to school. She was very nervous because she did not know how her classmates would react. But when she walked into her first-period class, "the students whistled and clapped and cheered, welcoming me back," she recalled.

"All morning, kids begged for a turn to carry my sticks up or down the stairs."[7]

The last class that day was chorus. Seven months after she first felt her leg muscles twitch, Peg was once again singing happily. She eventually graduated from high school, got married, and had two children. Not everyone who got polio, however, was as fortunate as Peg. Her friend Tommy whom she met at the polio hospital wound up in an iron lung. Tommy's polio had paralyzed his diaphragm, the muscle that controls breathing. An iron lung is a large, metal machine that does the breathing for a person with a paralyzed diaphragm. Shirley, another of Peg's hospital friends, died five years after getting polio.

Polio would continue to be feared until 1955. Doctors never developed a cure for polio. But that year an American doctor developed a way to protect people from getting polio. His name was Jonas Salk.

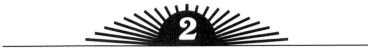

Survival and Success

IN 1916, DANIEL AND DORA SALK WERE afraid for their two-year-old son, Jonas. The family was living in Manhattan, one of the five boroughs that make up New York City. That year, a polio epidemic was sweeping across America. New York City was hit especially hard. Over 6,000 deaths from polio were reported that year in America. Of these, nearly 2,500 were New Yorkers. Most were children who were less than five years old.[1]

Starting in July that year, the front page of the *New York Times* reported the numbers of new polio cases and deaths. For a time, the New York Public Library closed its doors to children. People living in nearby communities tried to prevent New Yorkers from entering their towns and villages. Cars with children leaving New York City were turned back. The opening of public schools in the city was delayed for a month. New Yorkers, like Daniel and Dora Salk, were afraid for their children.

Daniel was a first generation American, born in New Jersey. His parents had come to America sometime in the late 1800s from Russia, where they had been the targets of religious prejudice. The Salks were Jewish. In Russia, Jews were forced to live in separate areas. They were not allowed to own land. Looking for a better life, the Salks decided to leave Russia and make a new home in the United States.

Dora was around twelve when she arrived in New York on a ship from Russia. She too was searching for a better life than was available to Jews in Russia. She did not speak English and was on her own. Soon after arriving in America, Dora got a job as a seamstress, sewing clothes in a factory and was made the forewoman of a team by the time she was fifteen.

When Daniel and Dora met, he was working

as a designer of lace patterns for women's blouses. They were married, and Jonas was born on October 28, 1914. Shortly after Jonas's birth, Dora stopped working as a seamstress and the family moved to an apartment in the Bronx—a borough of New York City. Here Jonas started elementary school. His mother had never attended school. His father had graduated only from elementary school. Still, his parents placed a high value on education.

Jonas' mother became the driving force in his young life. She was not satisfied with raising a smart and well-behaved child. She wanted more. As soon as Jonas measured up to her standards, she immediately raised those standards, always demanding more from her son.

As an adult, Jonas remembered that his "parents were more than supportive, my mother particularly. . . . She immediately, as a young girl, began to work to help support the family. And she was very ambitious, in a sense, for her children. [In addition to Jonas, the Salks would have two more sons, Herman and Lee.] She wanted to be sure that we all were going to

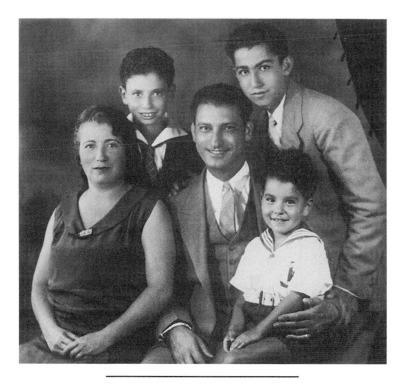

An early Salk family portrait circa 1931. Herman and Jonas Salk (left to right) stand behind their parents, Dora and Daniel. The Salks' youngest son, Lee, is seated on his father's lap.

advance in the world. Therefore we were encouraged in our studies, and overly protected in many ways." [3]

With his parents' support and encouragement, Jonas did very well in school. He learned quickly. Teachers were impressed with his curiosity. He always asked questions. As Jonas himself pointed out, "I think I was curious from the earliest age on. There was a photograph of me when I was a year old, and there was that look of curiosity on that infant's face. . . . I have the suspicion that this curiosity was very much a part of my early life: asking questions. . . . I tended to observe, and reflect, and wonder."[4]

In time, Jonas' parents had enough money to move to an even nicer apartment. This new home was in Brooklyn, another borough of New York City. This home was in an area where many successful Jewish families had settled after moving out of Manhattan's Lower East Side.

When he was twelve, Jonas was accepted by Townsend Harris High School. This was a public school that had been recently established for bright students from all over New York City. The school did not charge tuition, something that Jonas' parents appreciated. The students were warned that they would be expected to work hard, however. Every student had to finish the usual four years of high school in just three.

Townsend Harris High School did not emphasize science. While at the school, Jonas took only one science course—physics. He took this course not because he was interested in science, but rather because his friends were taking it. As Jonas admitted, "As a child I was not interested in science."[5] His interests in school were history and poetry.

Jonas graduated high school in 1929. In September of that year, he started college. He was three years younger than most students who were entering City College of New York that year. Jonas turned fifteen on October 28, 1929. The next day, the stock market crashed. America was about to enter the Great Depression of the

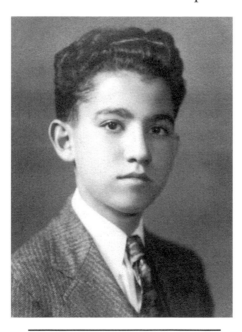

Jonas Salk is pictured here as a young teenager at Townsend Harris High School, approximately fifteen years old, circa 1929.

1930s. During this decade, many Americans suffered the worst poverty the country had ever faced. All over America, businesses failed. Banks closed. People begged.

As a teenager, Jonas faced more hardships than most people do in a lifetime. He was born into a family that had to work very hard just to survive. Disease and death were always a threat. The 1916 polio epidemic was not the only danger. In 1918, a flu epidemic killed more than 600,000 Americans.[6] In the 1930s, getting a job—even for a college graduate like Jonas— was almost impossible because of the Great Depression. Nonetheless, Jonas survived. In fact, he did more than survive—he succeeded. His first success was graduating near the top of his high school class when he was only fourteen. His next success would be college.

A Change of Plans

THROUGHOUT HIGH SCHOOL, JONAS wanted to become a lawyer. But after graduating, he changed his mind. As Jonas recalled, "My mother didn't think that I would make a very good lawyer, probably because I could never win an argument with her."[1] His mother was not the reason he decided to change his career plans, however. Rather it was his decision to try something different in college. Jonas signed up for some science courses. He liked them so much that he decided he wanted to become a scientist rather than a lawyer. Something else happened while Jonas was in college to spark his interest in science: the election of Franklin Delano

Roosevelt as president of the United States in 1932. Roosevelt was a polio survivor.

Roosevelt had caught polio in 1921. That August, Roosevelt, his wife, five children, and some friends were on vacation at their summer home in New Brunswick, Canada. After a day of boating and swimming, Roosevelt returned to the house to check his mail. As he sat in his wet bathing suit, he started to shiver. Rather than eat dinner, he went to bed with the hope that he would feel better in the morning.

However, the next morning, Roosevelt was in pain and had a high fever. Weeks passed. But the pain and fever remained. Finally, the doctors realized that Roosevelt had polio. He was thirty-nine years old. Now he could get around only by using a wheelchair. Years of therapy followed. He exercised, mostly swimming in warm, mineral water. In 1928, he was elected governor of New York. Four years later, he was elected president.

America had become fascinated with Roosevelt. His courage in fighting a paralyzing disease had inspired many people, including Jonas. By the time he was elected president,

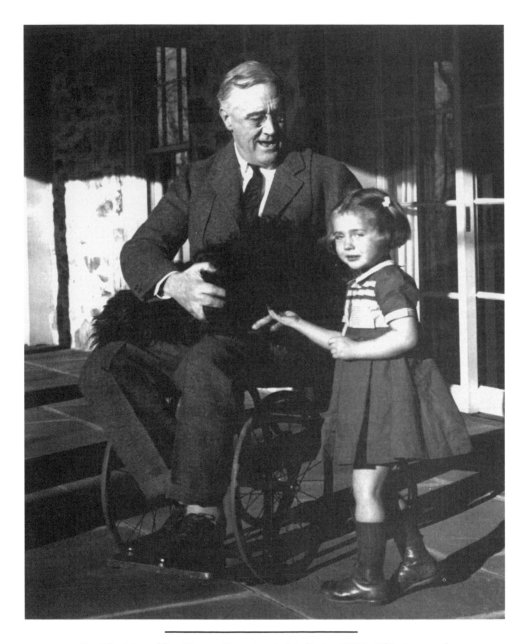

President Franklin Roosevelt contracted polio in 1921. This is one of the few photos in existence that show Roosevelt in his wheelchair.

Roosevelt had regained the use of many of his muscles. Only his lower legs and knees had to be supported by braces.

Jonas began to think about how he could make the world a better place. He decided to go to medical school. He started medical school when he was just about to turn twenty. In 1934, Salk entered New York University School of Medicine. College had not cost the Salks any money. The City College of New York did not charge students tuition. However, medical school was different. To help pay the tuition for his first year at medical school, Salk's parents took out a loan. In addition, he had saved money from his summer jobs. He had worked as a counselor in a boys' camp in the mountains north of New York City. While in medical school, he also earned scholarships and worked part-time jobs. His parents' loan, his savings, and his scholarships enabled Salk to pursue his medical studies.

After his first year of medical school, Salk took a year off. With the help of one his teachers, Salk had been granted a fellowship. A fellowship is a sum of money that is given to a person to study a particular area or subject. Salk decided to use his fellowship money to study bio-chemistry. This is the study of chemicals and how they react in living things, like humans. His study of biochemistry would be extremely useful to Salk in his later work.

After his year off, Salk returned to medical school. That year Salk took a course in micro-biology, which is the study of bacteria and viruses. Unlike viruses, bacteria are living things. Like all living things, bacteria take in nutrients, respond to changes in their environment, and reproduce. In contrast, viruses do not ingest anything and cannot reproduce by themselves. Instead viruses infect living cells where they take control and produce new viruses. Eventually all these viruses burst open the cell, killing it. The viruses can then infect other cells to continue their destructive cycle—unless they are somehow stopped.

But viruses and bacteria do have something in common. They are both extremely small and can cause disease. Salk learned how people could be protected against bacterial and viral diseases by a process called inoculation. An inoculation is an injection given to protect a person against a particular disease. Salk did not realize it at the time, but inoculation would be the means by which he would eventually conquer polio.

The use of inoculation to prevent disease was not new. In fact, its history can be traced back several centuries to China and India. At that time, many people died from a disease called smallpox. People with smallpox developed pus-filled blisters on their skin. Those who survived were left with deep scars on their skin. To protect against smallpox, a small amount of pus from a blister of a person with smallpox was scratched into the skin of a healthy person. But this procedure was risky. Although nine out of ten people developed only a mild form of the disease, one out of ten developed a severe case of smallpox. Many of these people died.

In 1796, an English doctor named Edward Jenner developed inoculation as an effective way to prevent smallpox. Jenner noticed that dairymaids (the women who milked cows) rarely got smallpox. Instead they got a related disease called cowpox. Cowpox was not nearly as serious as smallpox, and it rarely left scars. Jenner reasoned that cowpox somehow protected the dairymaids against smallpox. To test his idea, he inoculated a young boy with the pus from a cowpox blister instead of a smallpox blister. The boy developed cowpox. Months later, Jenner inoculated the boy with the pus from a smallpox blister. The boy never developed smallpox. The inoculation with cowpox had worked. Jenner called his process "vaccination," after the Latin word for cow (*vacca*). Most doctors and scientists ignored Jenner's work for more than fifty years. But by the time Salk was in medical school, vaccinations were routinely given to prevent several diseases, including the bacterial diseases diphtheria and tetanus.

Salk learned that bacterial vaccines could be prepared by treating the poisons made by bacteria, called toxins, with certain chemicals. These chemicals changed, or inactivated, the toxins so that they were no longer capable of causing disease. However, the body's immune system responded to these inactivated toxins as if they were still active. (The immune system is the body's main defense against germs that cause disease.)

Part of this defense involves white blood cells. These cells surround and destroy invading germs before they have a chance to do any harm. Once they have successfully done their job, these cells remain alert. If the germ again invades the body, these cells are ready to destroy it even more quickly the second time. These cells also respond to the treated toxins used in vaccines. The immune system is then prepared if the body is ever invaded by living bacteria of the same type.

Salk also studied viruses and the diseases they cause. He learned that vaccinations for viral diseases, such as smallpox, yellow fever, and rabies, were different from those used for bacterial diseases. Vaccinations could be developed using chemically-treated bacterial toxins. However, he was told that vaccinations could not be developed using chemically-treated viruses. Rather the person had to be vaccinated with a

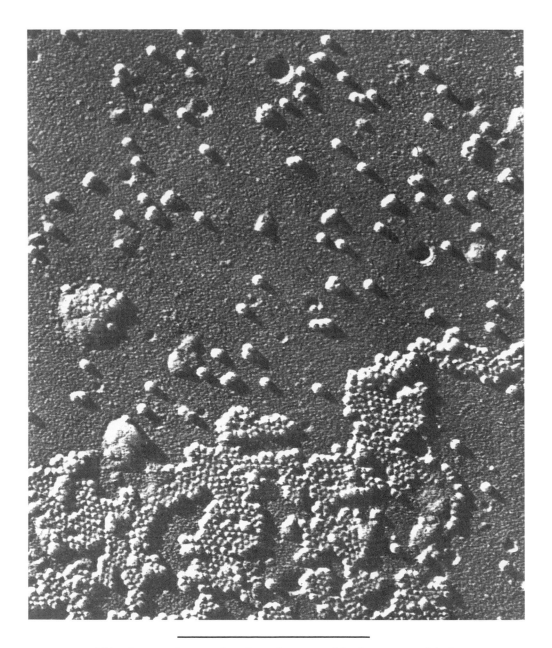

This photograph was taken through a powerful microscope and is the first image taken of the polioviruses.

small dose of a weakened form of a virus. In this case, the person might experience some symptoms of the disease. But these symptoms were usually mild and passed quickly. The person would then be protected against developing the viral disease later.

Salk also learned that there was a chance that a person vaccinated with a weakened virus might develop a full-blown case of the viral disease. This was rare, but it could happen. Salk and his fellow medical students were told that this risk was unavoidable.

Years later, Salk pointed out in an interview that he was confused when he first learned about vaccinations. "I asked why this was so. [Why vaccines could be developed with treated bacterial toxins but not with treated viruses.] There was no satisfactory answer."[2] Salk's curiosity had been aroused.

Not surprisingly, Salk did well in medical school. In his third year, he was elected to a society that honored those with high grades. By his fourth and final year, Salk was convinced that he wanted to become a research scientist rather than a practicing doctor. This was something that he had in mind when he entered medical school. He said so when he was interviewed for admission. At that time, the interviewer told Salk that he would not make as much money doing research. But Salk did not care. However, his parents did care, especially his mother. She dreamed of her son becoming a doctor and opening an office to treat patients. Salk, however, dreamed of doing research to find answers and solve problems, like diseases.

During their last year of medical school, students were given a two-month period during which they could study and work in an area that interested them. Salk hoped to spend this time studying various diseases at the Rockefeller Institute in New York City, but he was turned down. Salk then went to see Dr. Thomas Francis, who was doing research on viruses. Francis had just left the Rockefeller Institute, where he had been studying a virus that causes the flu, to work at New York University Medical School. Fortunately for both men, Francis welcomed Salk into his lab at the medical school.

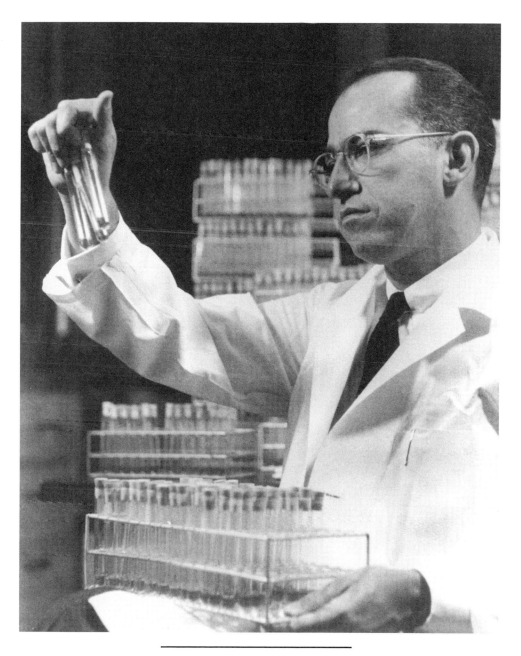

Jonas Salk is shown here at work in the laboratory.

Francis believed that vaccines could be prepared using treated viruses. Having asked himself the same question, Salk saw the value in this approach. He felt that he could learn a great deal about viral diseases and vaccinations from Francis. In turn, Francis looked at Salk as someone who would work hard and offer valuable ideas. Francis later said that Salk "seemed a good young man, interested, with ideas."[3]

Salk wasted no time in getting to work. Francis was interested in developing a vaccine against influenza. Influenza, or simply the flu, is caused by a virus. He had Salk remove the viruses from the lungs of mice who had been infected with the disease. Salk then treated the viruses with ultraviolet light and tested them to see if they were still active. Salk was able to publish a scientific paper with Francis. In it he described his research efforts. It would be the start of his lifelong work with viruses.

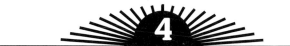

Relationships

SALK GRADUATED FROM MEDICAL SCHOOL
in June 1939. The day after his graduation, he
married Donna Lindsay. The two had been
engaged for a year. Their relationship would be
more than one between a husband and his wife.
Mrs. Salk was a social worker who specialized in
mental health counseling. As Salk put it, he was
"now ready to move forward in his career, with a
spouse who shared his intellectual interests and
goals of making the world a better place."[1]
Their relationship would last for almost twenty-
nine years.

His relationship with Dr. Francis also continued. After medical school, Salk went on
working in Francis' lab. Salk received a grant of

$100 a month from the Rockefeller Institute to carry out his research. (Grants are the main way scientists and doctors get money to support their research work.) In March 1940, Salk became an intern at New York City's Mount Sinai Hospital. That year, 250 medical students from all over the country had applied to be interns at Mount Sinai. Only eleven others, besides Salk, were accepted.

As an intern, Salk treated patients and attended lectures. The hours spent at the hospital were very long. Doing research work at Francis' lab made Salk's day even longer. A short time later, Francis left New York to head a virology lab at the University of Michigan. Salk remained at Mount Sinai. The two men, however, remained in close contact by letter.

Salk worked as an intern at Mount Sinai for two years. Once again, his efforts ended in success. His first year, he received the highest evaluations of any intern. His second year, he was given a position advising new interns. He was also elected president of the hospital housestaff by his fellow interns in recognition of his hard work. His work as an intern came to an

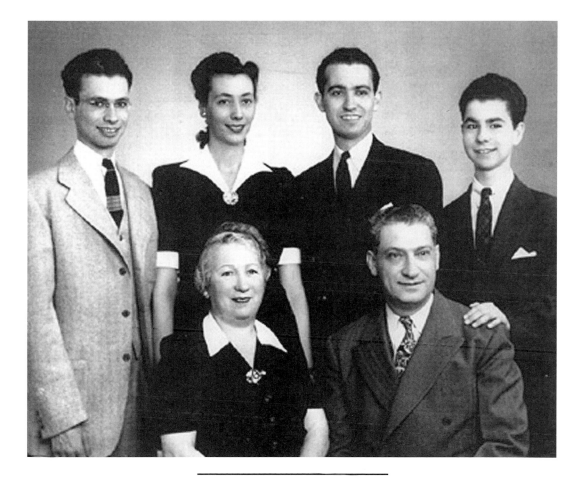

Newly-married Jonas Salk and his wife, Donna, are shown here in a family portrait with Herman Salk (far left), Lee Salk (far right), and Dora and Daniel Salk (seated), circa 1939.

end in 1942. Salk applied for jobs at several research institutes. Not one accepted him, most likely because he was Jewish. Salk refused to get discouraged. He wrote to Francis for advice.

Francis was amazed that no one would hire Salk. He immediately started looking for a way to bring Salk to the University of Michigan. He was able to scrape together enough grant money to offer Salk a job as his assistant. At this time, Francis was still working on the influenza virus. In fact, he was more involved in this work than he had been at Mount Sinai. In December 1941, the United States had entered World War II. The U.S. Army was most interested in getting an influenza vaccine. Army officers recalled the 1918 influenza epidemic that had killed hundreds of thousands of Americans. They feared that influenza could easily become an epidemic among the soldiers who lived in cramped barracks.

The money that Francis got for Salk came from a grant given by the army. The grant was for research on the influenza virus. It was enough to pay Salk $40 a week. It also kept him out of the army. Salk had been given until March

1, 1942 to either enlist in the army or be drafted. However, his work with influenza was so important that the government decided not to draft him.

In 1942, Salk and his wife left New York City for the University of Michigan. They rented a small farmhouse on the edge of town. Mrs. Salk got a job as a social worker. The Salks found life in Michigan very different from New York. They loved to take long walks in the countryside.

A visiting friend from New York wrote: "The last human being I expected to see using a wood-burning stove was Donna Salk, but there she was cooking on a wood-burning stove. And canning the produce raised in their huge vegetable patch."[2] While they were in Michigan, the Salks had two sons. Peter was born in 1944. Darrell was born in 1947.

Soon after his arrival in Michigan, Salk started his work on the influenza virus. This work proved very challenging. There are actually many different kinds of influenza viruses, called strains. Each strain is slightly different from the others. But they had one thing in common—they all could cause the flu. Salk and Francis realized that they had to isolate every strain of flu virus they could find. This was the only way to make an effective vaccine. If the vaccine did not contain all the strains, then the body would not be protected against those that were missing. But there were over 100 strains to check.

The next step was to find a way to destroy the viruses so that they could not cause the flu. They used a chemical called formaldehyde to inactivate the viruses, destroying their ability to cause disease. Although they are not considered living things, viruses that are inactivated are referred to as "killed viruses." Even though they have been "killed," these viruses must still be able to stimulate the immune system to be effective for use in a vaccine.

The final step was to prepare just the right combination of these killed viruses to make the vaccine. All these steps took a year to finish. Then in the winter of 1943, Salk and Francis were ready to test their vaccine.

About 2,500 soldiers were involved in the test.

Half of them got the vaccine. The other half got a placebo. A placebo is a substance that cannot help or harm a person. The group getting the placebo can then be compared to those getting the vaccine. To keep everything honest, neither the doctors nor the soldiers knew who was getting the vaccine and who was getting the placebo. If the vaccine worked, then those soldiers getting the vaccine should develop fewer cases of the flu than those soldiers getting the placebo. This is exactly what happened.

In the summer of 1944, 75 percent fewer cases of flu were reported among the soldiers who got the vaccine.[3] Salk and Francis had developed the first effective vaccine using treated viruses. As Salk later said, "I . . . developed a flu vaccine . . . that led to all sorts of other things."[4]

One of those things was a promotion. In 1946, Salk was made an assistant professor at the University of Michigan. What he really wanted though was to set up his own lab. This meant ending his working relationship with Francis. In 1947, Salk left the University of Michigan. He took his wife and two sons to the University of Pittsburgh School of Medicine.

Not long after his arrival in Pittsburgh, Salk wondered if he had made a mistake. His lab was rather small and in the basement of an old hospital. The first thing he had to do was clear out all the old furniture that had been stored there. Then he had to clean every inch of the lab. At the time, Pittsburgh was the center of the steel-making industry. Plants burned tons of coal to make the steel. Burning all this coal produced a lot of black soot. This soot covered everything in the city, including Salk's basement lab.

Salk also faced other problems. The city owned the hospital building where his lab was located. But as a member of the medical school faculty, the money for his research came from the university's science department. So whenever Salk wanted to buy something for his lab, he had to make out three separate requests. One went to the city, the second to the medical school, and the third to the science department. Only after all three parties had approved, did

Salk get what he wanted. Obviously, this took time that he could have spent doing research.

Although he was an associate professor, Salk was still not entirely on his own. He had to work under the direction of another doctor, who was in charge of the virus research program. This was a slight problem for Salk, who was interested in animal viruses. In contrast, the doctor in charge was working on plant viruses. Because they did not share the same interests, the two did not communicate as well as they could have.

Despite these problems, Salk realized he had made the right move. He finally had his own lab, where he continued working on the influenza virus. He soon discovered that adding certain substances to the flu vaccine made it even more useful. These substances made it possible to add more virus strains to the vaccine. Thus, a single vaccine could protect a person against more flu strains.

In 1948, Salk would welcome a visitor to his lab. The visitor, Dr. Harry Weaver, was the director of the National Foundation for Infantile Paralysis. (The term infantile paralysis is another

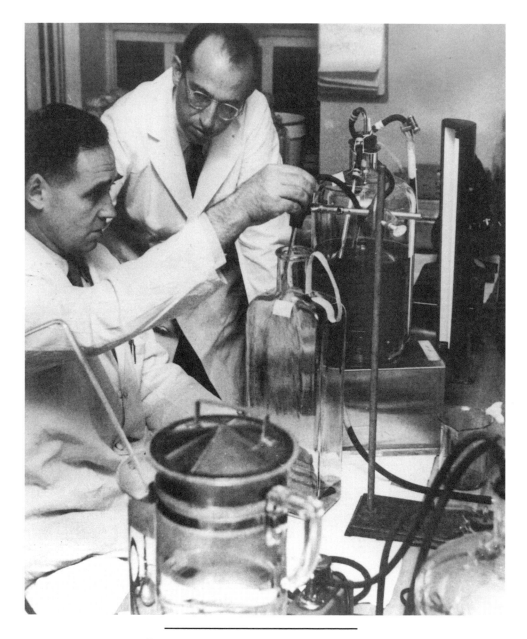

Dr. Jonas Salk (right) and Dr. P. L. Bazely are shown here at work in Salk's Pittsburgh laboratory.

way of saying polio. Infantile refers to the infants whom polio affected. Paralysis refers to the effect polio could have on the muscles of these children.) The National Foundation had been set up in 1937. President Roosevelt had played an important role in getting the foundation started. It had two purposes. One was to help treat polio victims. The other was to find a way to conquer polio. Salk did not realize it at the time, but his life would take a new direction because of Weaver's visit.

His Own Project

DURING HIS VISIT, WEAVER ASKED SALK IF he would be interested in working on the poliovirus. The first question that had to be answered was exactly how many different types of polioviruses there were. If a vaccine were to be effective, it had to protect people against all the types of polioviruses. At the time, scientists thought there were only three types. But no one was absolutely sure.

Salk agreed to work on the poliovirus. After all, it was a virus that was a serious threat to humans, just like the influenza virus. Besides, Weaver had promised Salk that he would get more lab space in the hospital. Salk would also get more laboratory workers. Most importantly, this would be Salk's own project. He could plan and carry out the experiments without needing anyone else's approval. His research would be supported by the March of Dimes.

The March of Dimes had its start in 1934. That year, President Roosevelt had his first birthday in office. He was fifty-two. Celebrations called Birthday Balls were held throughout the country in his honor. The main purpose was to raise money for a foundation that had been set up to fight polio. That first year, the Birthday Balls raised over one million dollars. More money was raised in the years that followed. But some people did not think that the president should be raising money for an organization, even one devoted to fighting a deadly disease.

As a result, the National Foundation for Infantile Paralysis was set up in 1937. Rather than having Birthday Balls to raise money, people were asked to contribute money to the new foundation. No amount was too small. Even a dime was welcomed. All the dimes that people gave might lead to an end of polio. The program would be called the March of Dimes. It began on Roosevelt's birthday that year,

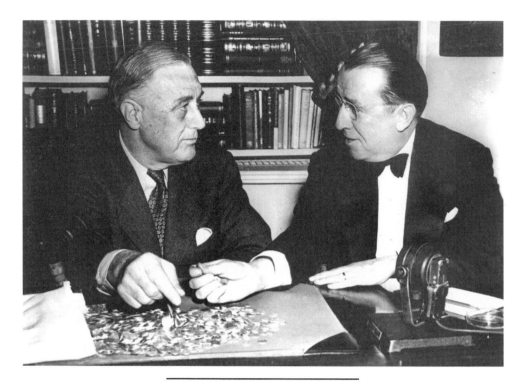

President Roosevelt (left) assists the head of the March of Dimes, Basil O'Connor, in counting a pile of donated dimes.

January 30, 1938. People from all over the country mailed their dimes to the White House. In its first year, the March of Dimes raised about $1.8 million. Much of this money was given to doctors and scientists working on the poliovirus. One of them would later be Salk.

But Salk was not the first to get money to carry out research on polio. In 1935, some of the money raised by the Birthday Balls went to Dr. Maurice Brodie to develop a vaccine. Brodie ground up the spinal cords of monkeys that had been given the poliovirus. He then added a chemical to kill the viruses that were in the mixture. After preparing a vaccine containing these killed viruses, Brodie next injected it into himself. He lived. Brodie then sought to inject his vaccine into children. He needed volunteers.

One of Brodie's fellow scientists volunteered his two sons. One of the boys wrote later in life: "At one point my brother and I, still young schoolboys, were whisked off . . . as reluctant volunteers . . . to receive large, painful intramuscular injections of the stuff."[1] Both boys lived. Brodie soon decided to test his vaccine on a large number of children. In California alone, some 1,600 children were injected with Brodie's polio vaccine in 1935. A number of these children died from the virus.[2] The use of Brodie's vaccine was stopped immediately.

That same year, Dr. John Kolmer also tested a polio vaccine. His vaccine was slightly different from Brodie's. Kolmer had tested his vaccine on monkeys—it seemed to work. He next decided to inject children with his vaccine. He also sent

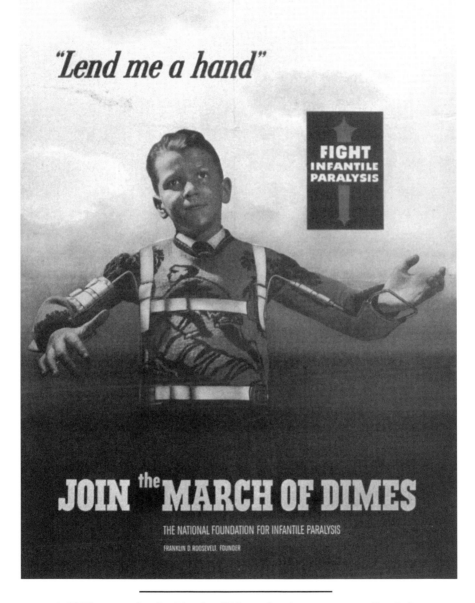

A 1951 poster for the March of Dimes showing a young polio victim fitted with arm braces.

his vaccine all over the country for doctors to use. The results were a disaster. Some of the children who were vaccinated became paralyzed. A few died.[3] The use of Kolmer's vaccine also came to a quick stop. People, including scientists and doctors, began to doubt that a safe polio vaccine could be developed. Salk was not one of those people.

Soon after Weaver's visit, Salk began his work on the poliovirus. By this time, scientists in other labs had discovered that there were at least three major types of polioviruses. Regardless of their type, polioviruses isolated from individual patients were each known as different strains. To find out if there were more than three major types of poliovirus, doctors decided to study more than 100 strains of polioviruses and determine into which type each strain belonged. This work would be very time consuming. Laboratories in two other universities shared the work with Salk.

At first, Salk had to use monkeys. Besides humans, monkeys are the only other living things that can develop polio. The plan Salk worked out was simple. He injected a monkey with a polio strain that he knew was type I. If the monkey's immune system overcame the virus, then Salk would inject a different strain.

If the monkey did not get polio, then the strain injected the second time was also type I. The immune system had recognized the virus injected the second time as being the same type that was injected the first time. As a result, the immune system quickly overcame the virus. The monkey did not get polio.

However, if the monkey got polio, then the strain injected the second time was not type I. In this case, the monkey's immune system had not been alerted. It had never before "seen" the virus injected the second time. Without the immune system to overcome it, the virus spread. The monkey got polio. Salk then had to do more tests to see whether this strain was type II, type III, or perhaps even a different type.

This process was very slow. More than 17,000 monkeys were used in these experiments. Salk had to wait months to see how each monkey did after an injection. If a monkey died from

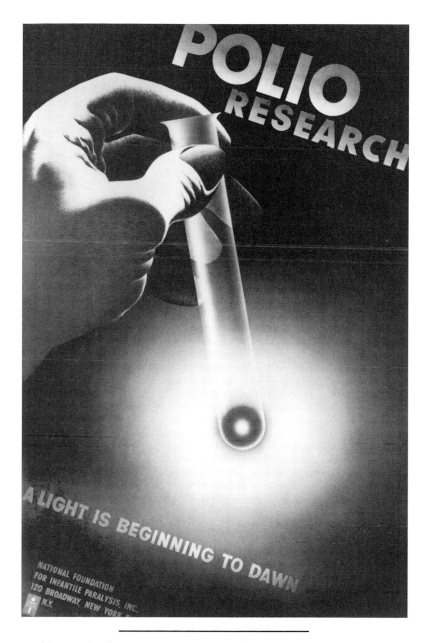

This March of Dimes poster promoted the positive strides being made in polio research during the early 1950s.

something other than the poliovirus, then the process would have to be repeated. Salk began to look for another way to speed up the process. But this would mean finding some way of growing the poliovirus outside of monkeys.

When Salk started working on the poliovirus, no one knew of a better method. Then in 1948, scientists at Harvard University found a way to grow the poliovirus outside a living animal. These scientists found a way to grow the virus in laboratory glassware containing cells and nutrients. Such a setup is called a tissue culture. Using tissue cultures to experiment with polioviruses would take much less time than using monkeys.

Unfortunately, the tissue culture method had not been developed when Salk was first working with polioviruses. As a result, it had taken Salk and the other two teams working on the project three years to place all the strains into one of the three types of poliovirus. The teams demonstrated that there were only the three types.

During those three years, and for the rest of his life, Salk worked very hard. "He just worked night and day," said John Troan, who was a science reporter for a Pittsburgh newspaper. Troan had met Salk shortly after his arrival at the University of Pittsburgh Medical School. In describing Salk's approach to work, Troan said, "He didn't like to fly at that time, and he would take a train overnight from Pittsburgh to New York. He'd work in New York, then he'd come back and I'd call his home. . . . And his wife would answer and say, 'You don't know Jonas, he went right to the lab.' And so he would be spending night and day there trying to get things going."[4] One of the things that Salk wanted to get going was a polio vaccine.

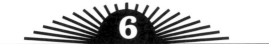

His Next Project

IN THE SPRING OF 1950, SALK WROTE TO Weaver to tell him that his next project was to find a way to vaccinate people against polio. One of his lab assistants recalled, "Salk says we've got these three types of viruses—what are we going to do with them? Why don't we make a vaccine that we can inject into animals, first, to see what's going on and then put them in people."[1]

In July 1950, Salk asked the National Foundation for more money. He wrote that the money would be used to find out if a polio vaccine could be developed for humans. His plan was to build upon the work that he and Francis had done with the influenza virus. Salk's idea was to develop a polio vaccine using killed viruses. Such a vaccine had been tested in monkeys by another scientist working on polio. The vaccine seemed to work, but it was not practical for human use because it was made using monkey cells. Salk realized that the new tissue culture techniques might allow him to develop a polio vaccine that would protect humans. In 1951, the National Foundation approved Salk's request for money. He was all set to begin working.

Salk killed each type of poliovirus separately with formaldehyde. He then made various combinations of the three killed virus types. Each combination was tested by injecting it into a healthy monkey. Salk then waited. What he was hoping for was that the monkey's immune system would respond to the vaccine. He would know this by examining a blood sample from the monkey.

If its immune system had responded, then the monkey's blood would contain antibodies against the poliovirus. (An antibody is a chemical that is made by a white blood cell when a virus or bacteria invades the body. Antibodies surround the invader until white blood cells can destroy it.) Salk soon discovered that the monkeys had developed antibodies against the killed viruses. Salk knew that the monkeys now had immunity against polio. Immunity means that an individual is protected against a particular disease.

Salk's polio vaccine seemed to work. Although the vaccine looked promising, many scientists doubted its value. They felt that the best approach to a polio vaccine was to use viruses that had been weakened but not killed. A weakened virus that can still reproduce and cause an infection is called an attenuated virus. They believed that an inoculation of attenuated viruses would give people more protection against polio. The most outspoken supporter of this approach was Dr. Albert Sabin, who was born in Russia, eight years before Jonas' birth in New York. Sabin immigrated to America as a young boy with his family. Like Salk, Sabin attended New York University Medical School. Following his graduation in 1931, Sabin's deep concern about the polio epidemics in New York City led him to focus his life's work on the poliovirus. For the rest of their lives, Sabin and Salk would find themselves at odds over the best way to conquer this disease. Each man would remain convinced that his was the best approach.

After his success with monkeys, Salk started to feel the pressure to begin testing his vaccine on humans. Part of this pressure came from the National Foundation, which had given Salk the money for his research. But Salk also put pressure on himself. In the early 1950s, new polio cases were rising rapidly. In 1948, there were about 27,000 new cases of polio. In 1950, the number of new cases climbed to near 33,000. In 1952, there were almost 59,000 new cases.[2] Obviously, something had to be done to stop the spread of polio. Not only America, but the whole world was becoming concerned about polio.

In September 1951, Salk traveled to Denmark to attend an international conference on polio. He had been chosen by the National Foundation to speak about his work on typing the viruses. Salk traveled by ship. On board were others heading for the conference. One of them was Sabin. The sea voyage would give everyone

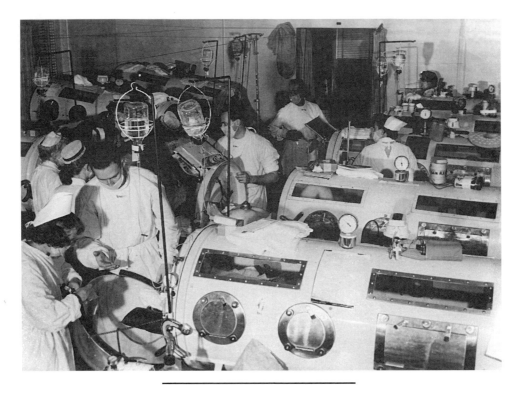

The emergency polio ward at Haynes Memorial Hospital in Boston, Massachusetts, is pictured here on August 16, 1955, as the city's polio epidemic hit a high of 480 cases. Critical patients are lined up close together in iron lungs so that doctors and nurses can give quick emergency treatment as needed.

time to talk about their work with polio. Sabin told Salk how he wanted to head a polio research institute. He suggested that the two might work together. Salk, however, was not interested. He did not want to give up the freedom to plan and carry out his own experiments.

At the conference, Salk spoke about how he

typed all the strains of poliovirus. He told the scientists that it was highly unlikely that more than three types of poliovirus would ever be found. Salk pointed out how much he owed to the scientists who had developed a way of growing the virus in tissue cultures. He emphasized his point by saying that a tissue culture started from one monkey could supply the same amount of virus that once took 200 monkeys.

Salk returned to America again by ship. During this voyage, he spent a good deal of time talking to Basil O'Connor. The two had met before, but they never had the time to talk at length. O'Connor was a close friend of President Roosevelt. When the National Foundation was set up, O'Connor became its first president. He had every reason to be interested in polio. Not only was his close friend President Roosevelt affected by it, but also his daughter. She came down with polio in 1950 and would be confined to a wheelchair for the rest of her life.

Salk and O'Connor found that they had more in common than an interest in polio. They had a

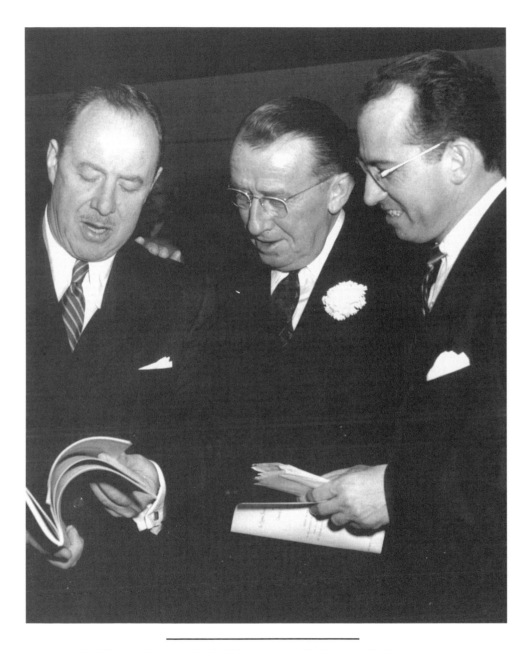

Dr. Thomas Francis, Basil O'Connor, and Dr. Jonas Salk (left to right) are shown together here in 1955.

mutual respect for each other. Both men had grown up in poverty. Both had succeeded through hard work. Most of all, both were determined to conquer polio. By the end of the voyage, O'Connor realized that if anyone could conquer polio, it was Salk. For his part, Salk was convinced that he could develop an effective vaccine within several years. Little did he know that he would be testing one sooner than that.

In December 1951, Salk attended another conference on polio. This one was held in New York City. By this time, Salk had started his vaccine experiments on monkeys. At the conference, he spoke about his belief that an effective polio vaccine could be made using killed viruses. In fact, another doctor at the conference reported that he had started using such a vaccine on children. He had injected six children with a vaccine containing killed viruses. Many of those at the conference expressed concern. The viruses had been grown in the spinal cords of monkeys. Doctors felt that this could cause an allergic reaction in the children.

Sabin was also present at the conference. As

he would for the rest of his life, Sabin spoke against Salk's proposal. Sabin said that the only way to make an effective polio vaccine was to use attenuated—not killed—viruses. Most scientists agreed with Sabin. Past experiments had shown that attenuated viruses produced an immunity that lasted longer. No one knew how long an immunity from a vaccine with killed viruses would last. But Salk would not be moved from his position. He and Sabin disagreed with each other every time they met. They had one thing in common, however: Each man wanted to conquer polio.

After the conference in New York City, Salk returned to his lab in Pittsburgh. He began to work harder than ever before. Not far from his basement lab was a constant reminder of what polio could do. On the fourth and fifth floors in the hospital above him were patients with polio. There were patients in wheelchairs. There were patients in iron lungs. And there were patients near death. Many were children.

Yet Salk knew that he had to take the time to be very careful. He was aware of the tests that

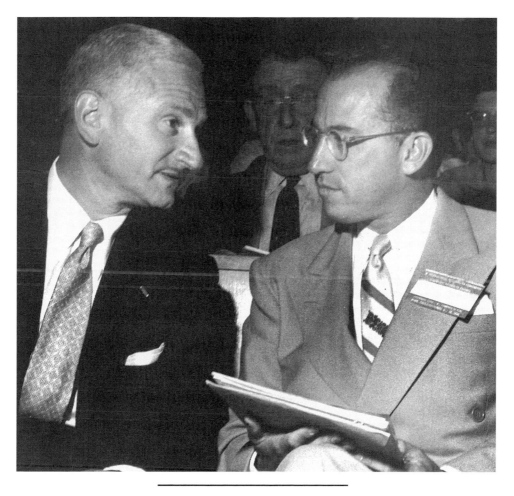

Dr. Albert Sabin (left) has a conversation with Dr. Jonas Salk.

others had already tried. He did not want his polio vaccine to paralyze or perhaps even kill someone. As Salk said, "I don't want to be rushed into anything. I want to take this step by step, just the way it should be done. Safety is first."[3]

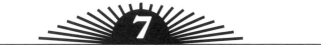

The Polio Vaccine

SALK SPENT ALMOST TWO YEARS developing his polio vaccine. During that time, he had actually developed several vaccines. Each had been made a different way. He tried different ways of growing the virus. He tried killing the viruses in different ways. He tried different combinations of killed viruses. All the vaccines were tested on monkeys. Finally in June 1952, Salk had a vaccine that he felt was safe to use on humans. The vaccine did not cause polio when injected into monkeys. The vaccine also stimulated the monkeys' blood systems to make antibodies against the virus.

Salk had decided who the first humans to receive his vaccine should be. They should be people who had been infected by the poliovirus and had recovered. These people would already have an immunity to polio. This way, there was little danger of them getting polio from the vaccine. Salk just had to make sure that each person got a vaccine with the same type of poliovirus that had infected them. Salk found such people at the D. T. Watson Home in a town near Pittsburgh.

The Watson Home was for children with disabilities. Many of them were paralyzed from polio. Salk selected forty children who were recovering from bouts with polio. On June 12, 1952, they were gathered together to begin testing the polio vaccine. First, Salk had to take blood samples from each of the children. He knew that the children already had antibodies against polio. Salk had to know exactly how much antibody each child had. What he hoped for was that his vaccine would increase the amount of antibodies in their blood.

The next month, Salk returned to the Watson Home. Like most vaccines, Salk's polio vaccine had to be injected into the arm. Some of the

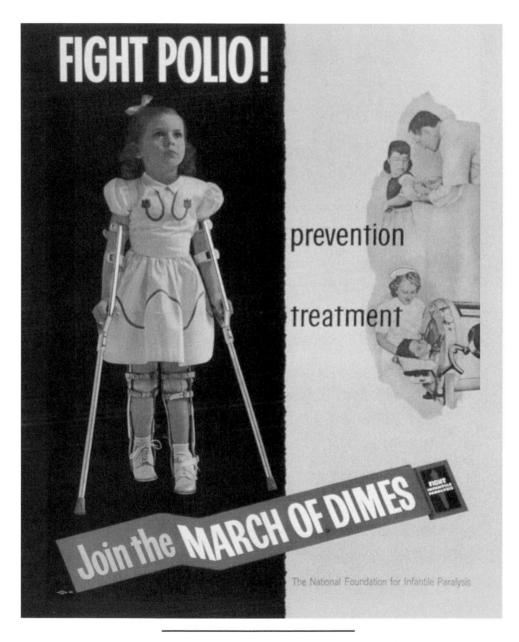

A 1955 poster for the March of Dimes showing a young polio victim fitted with leg braces and standing with metal crutches.

children were crying, in particular three very young ones at the head of the line. One of the young men who worked at the home came forward. His name was William Kirkpatrick. He volunteered to be the first to be injected to show the children that it did not hurt. On July 2, 1952, Kirkpatrick became the first person to be injected with Salk's polio vaccine. The forty children were next. That night, Salk returned to the home to check on each child. They were all fine. Still, he was concerned. As he later said, "When you inoculate children with a polio vaccine, you don't sleep well for two or three months."[1]

Salk's vaccine seemed to work. Blood samples taken from the children showed that they had developed more antibodies against the poliovirus. The vaccine boosted the immunity they already had. Salk knew what his next step had to be. He must inject his vaccine into people who did not have the same type of polio antibodies. Hopefully, they would develop antibodies against the new virus type and thus be protected from polio of the new type. Salk realized, however, that this test would be very different than the one he did on the children at the Watson Home. This time there was a chance that people could get polio from the vaccine.

Salk extended his study at the Watson home to include staff members and families of children with polio. He also went to another home to continue testing his vaccine. Called the Polk State School, this was a home for mentally retarded people. It was about 80 miles from Salk's home. Most of the residents had been placed in the Polk School shortly after birth. As a result, they had had very little contact with the outside world. It was likely that some of these individuals had never been exposed to the poliovirus. Blood samples were taken. They showed that some of the residents had no antibodies against the virus. Thus they had never been exposed to it.

Most of those Salk injected were in their teens and twenties. After getting the vaccine, they developed antibodies against the virus. Once again, Salk's vaccine seemed perfectly safe to give to humans. What's more, it seemed to

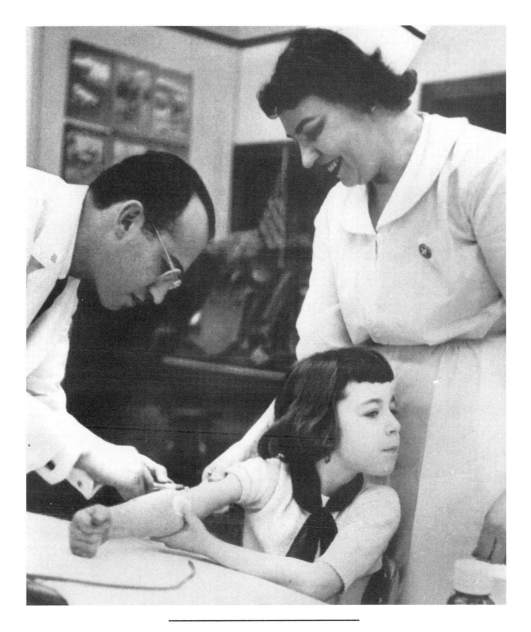

Dr. Jonas Salk injects a young girl with his polio vaccine during a field trial. Overall, 1,830,000 children participated in testing the Salk vaccine.

work. The antibodies the children had in their blood were enough to protect them from polio.

Salk next decided to give the vaccine to the workers in his lab. For years, they had been constantly exposed to the virus while working in the lab. Thus, their chances of developing polio were much higher than most people.

Next came Salk and his family. By this time, the Salks had another son, Jonathan, who had been born in 1950. Mrs. Salk recalled the day they were vaccinated: "I remember that the three kids and I were lined up in the kitchen. . . . I think he [Salk] gave it to himself first, he gave it to me, and he went down the line and gave it to the kids, and that was all. . . . And it really didn't occur to me [that] this is a historic moment."[2]

Salk's tests had been kept secret. The only ones who knew about them were Salk, his co-workers, those at the Watson Home and the Polk School, and a few people at the National Foundation. Salk did not want publicity and did not want people to expect too much, too soon.

Today, Salk would not have been able to carry out these tests without first getting government approval. Strict regulations by various agencies of the government now require that they review and approve the use of any drug or vaccine in humans for the first time. The drug or vaccine must first be tested on animals, such as mice, rats, and monkeys. If these animals do not develop any serious problems, then the drug or vaccine can be tested on a group of humans who have volunteered to participate in the test. Although Salk had adhered to all these precautions, it was not until many years later that the government required review and approval of all the details of these steps.

In January 1953, Salk attended a National Foundation conference on polio. There he presented a paper titled "Studies in Human Subjects on Active Immunization Against Poliomyelitis." (Poliomyelitis is the full, scientific name for polio.) Salk told how he had prepared a vaccine using killed viruses. He reported on the success of his experiments. Most of those present immediately began to wonder if a much larger test should be done. Salk, however, did not have enough vaccine to carry out such a test.

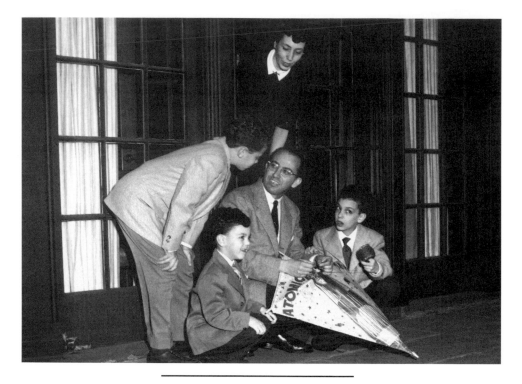

This 1955 photo shows Jonas Salk helping his three sons assemble a kite while Donna Salk looks on. From left to right are Peter (age eleven), Jonathan (age five), and Darrell (age eight).

In February, Salk attended a special meeting on polio in New York City. Again he explained what he had done. He reported that the details of his experiments were going to be published the following month. They would appear in the *Journal of the American Medical Association*, a leading publication for doctors and scientists. Word of Salk's success would soon spread throughout the world of science. But word got out even sooner than Salk expected. A newspaper article came out before his paper was published. The newspaper headline read "New Polio Vaccine—Big Hopes Seen."[3]

Salk was furious. He realized that people across the country would soon be demanding that their children get the vaccine. But there was no vaccine for use on the public. His experimental vaccine had not been fully tested, and there was not enough to give everyone. Salk thought it was best to speak to the American public directly. On March 26, 1953, Salk gave a nationwide radio speech called "The Scientist Speaks for Himself."

During his speech, Salk described the research work he had done on polio. He explained how the virus caused paralysis. He went on to talk about his vaccine. At the end of his speech, he warned the American people that it was not possible to prepare enough vaccine before the next polio epidemic that summer. Salk appealed for people to be patient. But he promised that "we can now move forward more rapidly and with more confidence."[4]

Despite the successful results, scientists were still concerned about Salk's vaccine. No one knew, for example, how long the immunity would last. If it did not last very long, then people would have a false sense of security, thinking they were protected from polio when they really were not. Scientists were also concerned that the vaccine might interfere with a person's immune system. This might make the person more likely to develop bacterial and viral diseases, including polio. Once again, Sabin was among those who argued strongly against Salk's vaccine. In part, Sabin felt that an effective vaccine could be made only by using a live virus. Sabin also appeared to be reacting as a competitor in a race for a polio vaccine.

The National Foundation, however, thought it wise to test Salk's vaccine on a much wider scale. The only way to know if the vaccine worked was to give it to large numbers of children in an area where a polio epidemic was likely to occur the following summer. One of Salk's biggest supporters at the National Foundation was Basil O'Connor. Their relationship had continued since they first talked during their return voyage from Denmark two years earlier. O'Connor was careful not to give the impression that the foundation was favoring Salk. The foundation was also giving money to Sabin and others for work on polio vaccines using attenuated viruses.

The months following Salk's radio speech were very hectic. Salk was still trying different combinations and ways of killing the virus to make the most powerful vaccine possible. He was also working with drug companies. Salk's lab would never be able to produce enough vaccine to inject tens of thousands of children. It would have to be made by drug companies. However, he did not want just one company making the vaccine. In his mind, that would be unfair because all the profits would go to just that one drug company. Instead, Salk wanted several companies to be involved. Every drug company though would have to follow his method for making the vaccine. This would not be easy. Making huge amounts of the vaccine in a large company was not the same as making a small amount in a lab.

A lot of time was also spent on planning how to carry out the test. Everyone knew that tens of thousands of children had to be injected with the vaccine. But how would these children be chosen? How would all these records be kept? How would everyone involved be kept honest? Most importantly, how would they know for sure that the vaccine worked? Several proposals were made. Salk, however, did not like any of them.

For a time, it looked as if the test would never be done. Fortunately, someone was found to supervise the test and make sure it was done honestly. That person was Dr. Thomas Francis. Salk and Francis knew each other since they had first met in New York City fifteen years earlier. Salk respected Francis and trusted him to perform a careful, scientifically correct study.

The Polio Pioneers

FRANCIS ARRANGED FOR A DOUBLE-BLIND test. This involves two groups. One is called the experimental group. Those in this group get the treatment. The other is called a control group. Those in this group get a placebo. In a double-blind test, no one knows who is in the experimental group and who is in the control group. This includes both the volunteers in the study and the doctors. Thus, the volunteers are "blind" because they do not know whether they are getting the treatment or a placebo. The doctors are also "blind" because they do not know whether they are giving the treatment or the placebo.

Francis also arranged that all the results

would be sent to him at the University of Michigan. He told everyone involved, including Salk, that he would not give out any information until he was ready. Everything was all set. What would be the largest scientific study ever done was about to begin. However, some people were trying hard to stop it. Sabin was one. He went to Washington, D.C. to testify before Congress. He warned that it was unsafe to give children a vaccine using killed viruses. He even wrote to Salk, telling him that it would ruin his career if the study went ahead. Not surprisingly, Salk moved ahead. Still, he was fully aware that "millions of lives were at risk."[1]

On February 23, 1954, the study began when Salk himself injected 137 children in a school in Pittsburgh. That spring and summer, 1.8 million schoolchildren would be involved in the polio study. Some would get the vaccine. Some would get a placebo. Still others would get nothing. These children would simply be observed to monitor their health. Some 20,000 doctors, 40,000 nurses, 50,000 teachers, and 200,000 volunteers participated in the study. These volunteers did various jobs. Many spoke to parents to get their permission to have their child be part of the study. Others set up places where the children could get injected. Some kept track of the results that were eventually sent to Francis.

Everyone knew that the study would take time. The children had to be injected three times. For those getting the vaccine, the first injection was meant to stimulate the making of antibodies against the poliovirus. After their first injection, each child got a button that said "Polio Pioneer." The second and third injections were meant to make the immune system form even more antibodies. Salk believed that this would give the children immunity against polio that would last. Blood samples also had to be taken from each child to keep track of their antibody levels.

Even before the results were known, people started talking about the "Salk vaccine." In reporting how the study was going, newspapers also called it the "Salk vaccine." Rather than welcome the attention, Salk told people that the

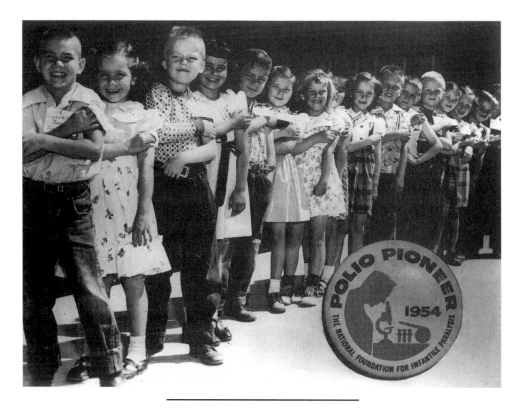

Young "Polio Pioneers" are shown here shortly after receiving their vaccinations in 1954.

vaccine should not be named after just one individual. "It embarrasses me . . . to have it called [the] 'Salk vaccine.' I'm not entitled to that kind of credit."[2]

Salk pointed out that his vaccine was the result of the work of many scientists. He reminded everyone that he had learned much from what others had discovered about the poliovirus. If anything, a friend of Salk suggested, it should be called the "Pitt vaccine."[3] This would honor the University of Pittsburgh Medical School where Salk first started working on polio. Despite these concerns, it would always be popularly known as the Salk vaccine.

Finally, Francis thought he had enough information to make an announcement. On April 12, 1955, he reported the results to the American public. Hundreds of scientists and doctors had gathered at the University of Michigan to hear what Francis was going to say. There were even more reporters present. Obviously, Salk was also there, along with his wife and three sons.

Francis had prepared a 128-page paper. It reported how the vaccine had done against the three types of polio. Francis told the audience that the vaccine was 60 to 70 percent effective against the type I virus and 90 percent effective against types II and III. Overall, he reported that the double-blind tests showed the vaccine to be 80 to 90 percent effective against polio. Newspaper reporters jumped on the story.

Headlines that day read "VICTORY OVER POLIO! POLIO VACCINE WORKS!"[4]

When Francis finished his report, Salk got up to speak. Everyone in the audience stood up and clapped. Salk then talked about his work. He went on to tell the people how he planned to make the vaccine 100 percent effective. He had ideas for making a more powerful vaccine. He also thought it best to give the second injection two to four weeks after the first. The third injection would be given seven months later. Salk said that he felt this schedule would best prepare the immune system against polio. But some people in the audience were annoyed about Salk's comments. They felt that he should not be talking about a vaccine that had yet to be developed and a schedule that had yet to be worked out.

Shortly after Salk had finished speaking, government officials gathered to discuss a nationwide vaccination of school children. Just hours after Salk's speech, the federal government issued a license so that drug companies could begin shipping the vaccine. With financial

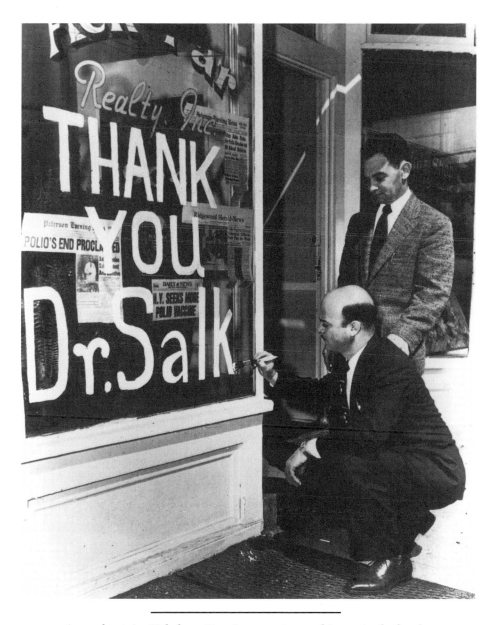

A merchant in Hohokus, New Jersey, expresses his gratitude for the Salk vaccine with this painted message on his store window shortly after the vaccine was announced as effective.

support from the National Foundation, several companies had made large quantities of the vaccine even before Francis gave his report. As a result, they were ready to supply doctors all over the country with the vaccine. The campaign to stop polio was underway.

Then tragedy struck. Two weeks after the nationwide program began, a child who had been vaccinated developed polio. The next day, five more vaccinated children came down with polio. Eventually, 260 people developed polio after getting the Salk vaccine. Of these, eleven would die.[5] Suddenly, the Salk vaccine seemed more of a health threat than a medical miracle. On May 7, 1955, all polio vaccinations were stopped. This was less than a month after Francis had reported how well the vaccine worked. Salk told reporters that a thorough investigation would have to be made.

Scientists immediately starting looking for answers. Their search led them to one of the drug companies making the vaccine, called Cutter Laboratories. They had discovered that all those who developed polio had been given a vaccine made at this lab. When they examined samples of the vaccine, they discovered that it contained live viruses. The lab had not followed Salk's detailed instructions for making the vaccine.

New rules were set in place. Drug companies had to take extra steps to make sure that their vaccines did not contain live viruses. The companies also had to report to the government on all the batches of vaccine they made. This way the government could be sure that Salk's directions were being strictly followed. On May 27, the government announced that the polio vaccination program could start again.

From the beginning, Salk had never sought to make money on his vaccine. He felt that it belonged to the people. But obviously, it would cost money to make the vaccine and inject it into millions of children. O'Connor had used National Foundation money to buy large supplies of the vaccine. His plan was to give it out free. Trained volunteers could inject the vaccine. The government, however, would not go along with O'Connor's idea. They feared that the public would then expect the government to

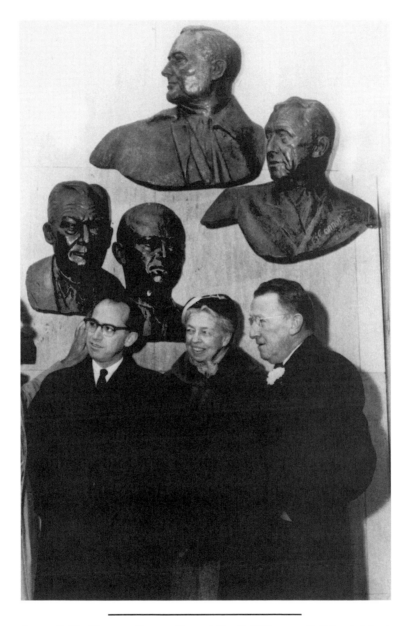

Jonas Salk, Eleanor Roosevelt, and Basil O'Connor (left to right) at the Infantile Paralysis Wall of Fame in Warm Springs, Georgia, on January 2, 1958.

pay for vaccines for all kinds of diseases. People simply had to pay for the vaccine. For those who could not afford it, the government set up a fund of $30 million.

In 1956, only 15,140 new polio cases were reported in America, reducing the number of polio cases by about 60 percent in just two years.[6] The Salk vaccine had stopped the spread of polio. By 1961, the number of cases of polio was reduced by more than 90 percent.[7]

For years, Sabin had argued that a polio vaccine could only be effective if it were made from attenuated viruses. In 1962, such a vaccine developed by Sabin and tested in Russia was introduced in the United States. Gradually, the Salk vaccine was being given less and less. Sabin claimed that his vaccine had three major advantages. It was easier and less expensive to make. It could be taken by mouth in a liquid dropped on a sugar cube. It provided a stronger, longer lasting immunity.

By the late 1960s, only the Sabin vaccine was being widely used in the United States. Several other countries continued to use only Salk's vaccine because they did not believe Sabin's claims. Salk was not surprised by Sabin's behavior. Salk once commented "I remember in Copenhagen in 1960, [Sabin] said to me, just like that, that he was out to kill the killed vaccine."[8]

Despite what later happened to his vaccine, Salk became an American hero the day Francis gave his report on April 12, 1955. His son Darrell told what happened after his father had spoken that day: "There were newspaper people around, there were cameras, and . . . this was really neat. We ended up getting a police escort on the way home . . . and it was a great thrill, very exciting. Better than a roller coaster."[9] Salk's own life certainly became much more like a roller coaster ride.

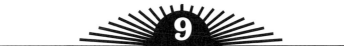

9

An American Hero

THE DAY FRANCIS GAVE HIS REPORT, Salk's picture appeared in newspapers all across America. That night, Salk appeared on a television show called *See It Now*. At the time, this was the most popular television news show, watched by millions of Americans. People finally got the chance to see what their hero looked like. He was a tall, thin man with glasses. To most people, Salk looked exactly like a scientist in the movies. But people could not help but be impressed by what they heard that night.

On the show, Salk once again reminded people that he owed his success to what other scientists had done before him. In fact, he pointed out that the history of the polio vaccine could be traced back to the 1860s with the work of the French scientist Louis Pasteur. It was Pasteur who had first convinced the world that germs can cause disease. As he had said many times before, Salk repeated that "this is not the Salk vaccine. This is a poliomyelitis vaccine."[1] He expressed his hope that everyone in America would soon benefit from the vaccine. As he put it, he would like a vaccination program to start immediately that would give "everyone some hamburger, instead of sirloin steak to a few."[2] In other words, the vaccine should be made available, either free or at little cost, to everyone.

The Salks had planned to stay in Michigan only two nights. All Salk wanted to do was hear Francis' report. The Salks wound up spending five days in Michigan. During that time, their phone would not stop ringing. Calls were coming in from all over the world. Mail started arriving in sacks. Some contained checks and money orders to help pay for the cost of producing the vaccine. Magazine and news-paper reporters wanted to write stories about the now-famous family.

When the Salks finally did return to Pittsburgh, they found a crowd waiting at the airport. There was also a police guard at their front door. The calls and the mail followed them from Michigan. If anything, it got worse. The Salks had to get an unlisted telephone number. The amount of mail they received grew each day. Many of the letters were from children. Teachers across the country were having their students write thank-you letters to Salk. Some were from children who discovered that they had received the placebo in the vaccine test. Now these children were saying they could not wait to get the "real thing."

Hollywood was also calling Salk. All the major studios wanted to do a movie about his life. Salk refused their proposals. He would accept only if the story were true and all the profits went to the research on polio.

Salk received invitations to speak all over the country. The first year following Francis' report, Salk made nearly eighty speeches. He was also asked to be the guest of honor at dinners where he would be given an award. He refused most of them. One he did accept was from President Dwight D. Eisenhower. At first, Salk did not even want to go. He was finding that all the attention he was getting was beginning to interfere with his work. But he realized that he could not turn down an invitation from the president. The two men met just seven days after Francis' report. Eisenhower told Salk in a voice filled with emotion, "I have no words to thank you. I am very, very happy."[3] As a grandfather, Eisenhower realized how valuable a contribution Salk had made.

Salk was certainly at the top of his roller coaster ride. But it was soon to head downhill fast. Four days after his meeting with the president, Salk had to face the problem of the deaths caused by the Cutter Labs vaccine. Once the problem was solved, Salk's ride took another turn uphill. While his vaccine was being tested, Salk was offered a promotion. The University of Pittsburgh wanted him to head a new department. But after thinking about it, Salk declined. He did not want to give up the chance to work in his lab every day.

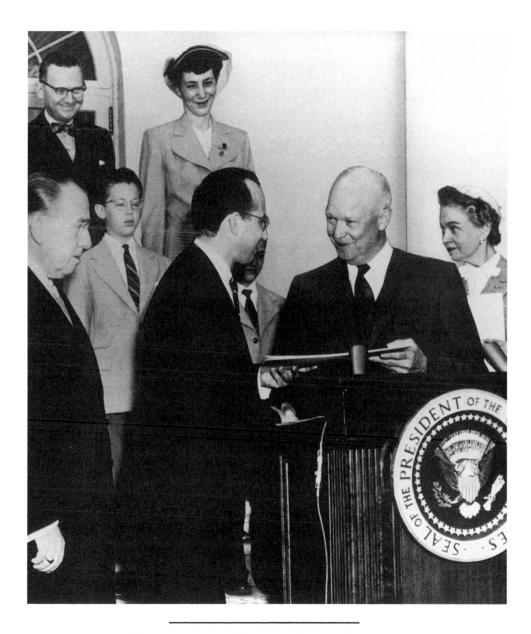

Jonas Salk receives an award from President Eisenhower on the White House grounds on April 22, 1955. Salk's wife and children look on while Basil O'Connor stands directly behind him.

The university then made him another offer. Money had been raised to buy the hospital building where Salk had his lab. In 1957, the building was turned over to the university and renamed Salk Hall. Here Salk would have total control in carrying out his research work. His work, however, never got started. The University of Pittsburgh had brought in a new president. He was not willing to allow Salk total freedom to do whatever he wanted. Rather, he wanted Salk to submit his plans for approval. This was something Salk was unwilling to do. Both men knew that the time for Salk to leave Pittsburgh was near.

Salk was also facing new problems with his vaccine. Two months after Francis' report in 1955, the American Medical Association (AMA) went on record against the use of his vaccine in public clinics. They wanted only private doctors to administer the vaccine in their offices. Despite these problems, 10 million children were vaccinated in 1955. As more vaccine became available in the following years, Salk personally appealed to people to get vaccinated.

By 1957, more than half of all Americans under the age of forty had been vaccinated.[4] By 1962, only 910 new cases of polio were reported.[5] Once again, Salk was on top—but not for long.

That year, Sabin's vaccine was approved for use by the government. It had been recommended by the AMA the year before. From then on, use of the Salk vaccine declined in the United States. But by 1963, Salk had moved on to other things. The Salk Institute for Biological Studies, near San Diego, California, opened that year. Salk had attracted some of the best scientists in the world to work at his institute. As Salk put it, the scientists at the institute should be "interested not only in science but in the whole range . . . of man's life."[6] The institute quickly became the center of Salk's life.

At the institute, most of Salk's work focused on cancer and multiple sclerosis, which is a disease of the brain and nerves. During his earlier work with viral diseases, Salk had become interested in how the immune system works. He had discovered that certain cancer cells grow in monkeys with an abnormal immune system, but not in monkeys with a normal, functioning immune system. Salk reasoned that cancer might be a disease in which the immune system failed to protect against cancer cells. He then began to investigate a disease in guinea pigs that was similar to multiple sclerosis in humans. In this disease, the immune system attacks normal nerve cells.

Salk wondered how the immune system could cause cancer by not working well enough and also could cause multiple sclerosis by working "too well." Instead of investigating germs and poisons that come from outside the body, Salk asked questions about how the body worked to cause disease. He once again was looking at a problem from a different point of view than most of his colleagues.

Over the years, fame took its toll. Salk had to spend long periods of time away from his family. In 1968, Jonas and Donna Salk separated after twenty-nine years of marriage. In 1970, Salk married Françoise Gilot. The two met while she was visiting the institute. Once the two

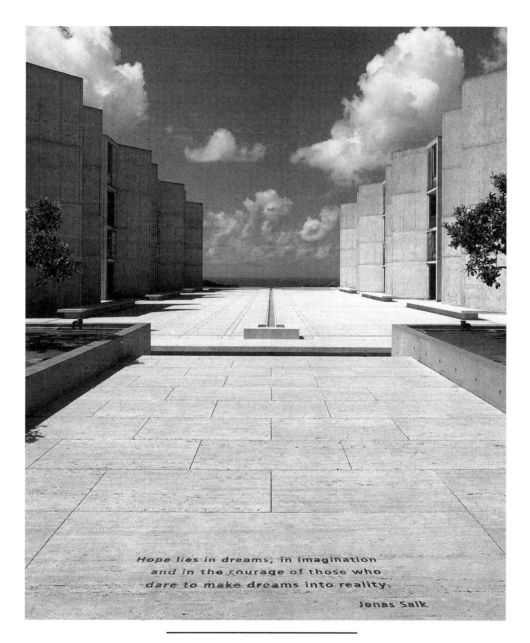

The courtyard entrance to The Salk Institute for Biological Studies in
La Jolla, California.

announced their engagement, the media would not give them any privacy. Salk and Gilot went to Paris to be married. In order to keep the wedding private, they got married the day before the announced date. After their honeymoon, they set up their new home near the institute where Salk continued to work. Salk would have a laboratory at the institute until 1984 and would work there for the rest of his life.

Shortly after his marriage to Gilot, Salk turned his attention to writing. In 1972, he published his first book, *Man Unfolding*. This book was followed by three others. Salk's books dealt with how science was affecting humankind. These books were not meant for scientists but rather for the general public. Salk wanted people to be aware of how drastically their lives could change because of science.

Salk published his last book in 1983. That same year, he turned his attention to AIDS. AIDS is the final stage of disease that develops after someone becomes infected with the virus known as HIV (human immunodeficiency virus).

The disease was first identified in 1981 in the United States, but researchers have traced cases back to as early as 1959. AIDS began to grow widespread in the 1980s and continues to be a deadly threat today: since the beginning of the epidemic through the end of 2001, it is estimated that 21.8 million total deaths have occurred worldwide as a result of AIDS.[7]

The name AIDS (which stands for "Acquired Immune Deficiency Syndrome") refers to the fact that HIV severely damages a person's immune system. The person can then get all kinds of infections, many of which are deadly without a working immune system. After the HIV damages the immune system enough, patients may develop skin lesions, pneumonia, and weight loss, among other symptoms. Eventually, these symptoms become classified as AIDS. Some people may become infected with HIV and carry it for several years before actually developing any symptoms. So it is possible for someone to be HIV-positive (carry the virus) without having AIDS.

Although Salk wanted to develop a vaccine to prevent infection—the way most vaccines work and the way his polio vaccine had worked—he knew that it would be very difficult to get approval to test a vaccine on unexposed (HIV-negative) persons. So instead he considered the incubation period (the time between when HIV is contracted and AIDS develops) in HIV-positive people. This led him to realize that an HIV vaccine could be used therapeutically, after virus infection had occurred. In this fashion, the vaccine might boost the immune system enough so that AIDS would not develop.

In 1992, Salk attended an AIDS conference in Europe. In a speech, Salk announced that he would be taking a new approach to fighting AIDS: Instead of using his vaccine to prevent infection with HIV, he would use it to prevent the development of AIDS in patients who were already HIV-positive.

His talk confused and angered some of those who were listening. But Salk had always spoken his mind. He never hesitated to go against what most others believed. This may be the reason why Salk never received praise from many of his fellow scientists. They never invited Salk to join

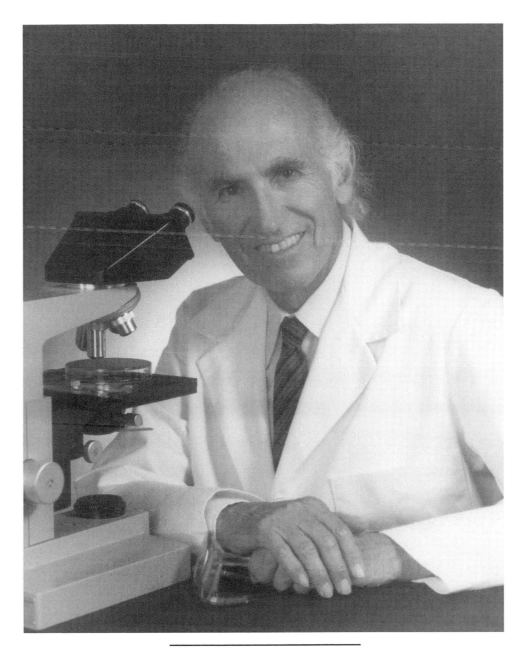

Dr. Jonas Salk is pictured here circa 1990.

the National Academy of Sciences, although Sabin was.

Salk's failure to win the respect of his fellow scientists may have started right after the success of his polio vaccine was first announced in 1955. The March of Dimes pushed Salk into the spotlight. Their hope was that the publicity would mean more money for the National Foundation. But many of Salk's fellow scientists resented all the publicity he was getting.[8] Despite how he and others felt about his fame, it would stay with Salk the rest of his life.

Jonas Salk died on June 23, 1995, at the age of eighty. The cause of death was heart failure. Salk once said in an interview, "You never have an idea of what you might accomplish. All that you do is you pursue a question and see where it leads."[9] The question he asked himself in medical school about vaccinations using treated viruses led Jonas Salk to his victory over polio.

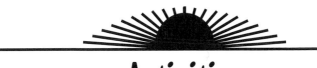

Activities

In Salk's Footsteps

Thanks first to Salk and then to Sabin, polio is no longer a health threat—at least in most parts of the world. The last reported case of an American getting polio through contact with the virus was in 1979. In 1993, the total number of polio cases reported in the world was about 100,000. Most of these cases occurred in Asia and Africa. In 2000, the Global Polio Eradication Organization set a goal to eliminate the disease worldwide by 2005.[1]

Even if polio is wiped out in every corner of the world, it will still leave its mark on humans. In the United States, there are an estimated 600,000 survivors of polio. Worldwide there are thought to be as many as 20 million survivors. At one time, doctors believed that anyone who overcame their polio paralysis could expect to live a normal life.

However, in the 1970s doctors first began hearing complaints from polio survivors. Many of them started to report muscle pain and weakness, a feeling of tiredness, sleeping problems, and trouble swallowing and breathing. Doctors questioned whether these people were suffering from delayed effects of a polio infection that they had some twenty, thirty, or even forty years earlier. Today, doctors recognize what is known as "post-polio syndrome." These are symptoms that polio survivors can experience many years after they were first infected by the virus.

A Tricky Virus

Consider what happened to Lauro Halstead. He got polio in 1954 when he was eighteen and had just finished his first year of college. When his diaphragm became paralyzed, Halstead was placed in an iron lung. Gradually, he regained the use of his muscles. Although his right arm remained paralyzed, he resumed a normal life and graduated college. Three years after getting polio, Halstead climbed Mount Fuji in Japan. When he reached the top, he thought to himself, "Polio is behind me. I have finally conquered it."[2]

But the poliovirus is quite tricky. For most people, the poliovirus does not cause any damage and simply passes out the intestines. For others, the poliovirus may cause paralysis that can be fatal. For those who overcome their paralysis, the poliovirus may show its effects many years later. How can all this be the work of one virus? The answer lies inside its protective covering.

A Recipe for Nucleic Acid

Viruses are simple. They are made of only two types of chemicals. One is a protein and makes up a virus' outer layer. The other is a nucleic acid and is found inside the protein layer. Nucleic acid stores the information that all living things, even viruses, need to function. Although this information can be very complex, getting the nucleic acid out of cells is simple. Here is one way to do it.

Place about 100 milliliters (ml) of green split

peas, a large pinch of table salt, and about 200 ml of cold water in a blender. Turn on the blender to high for twenty seconds. You now have cold pea soup. Filter this pea soup through a strainer into a clean container. Add two to three tablespoons of a liquid detergent to the filtered pea soup. Use the spoon to gently stir the soup and detergent. Let it stand for fifteen minutes.

Pour some of the pea soup into a small glass container. Add a pinch of meat tenderizer to the pea soup. Stir very gently. Tilt the glass container. Carefully pour rubbing alcohol down the side of the container. The alcohol should form a layer on top of the pea soup. Add about as much alcohol as you have pea soup. Use a thin wooden skewer to stir the liquids where the two layers meet. A whitish, stringy material should start to collect around the skewer. This is a nucleic acid. You can experiment by trying to get the nucleic acid from onions, spinach, and broccoli. Which gives you the most nucleic acid?

The nucleic acid inside the poliovirus has the information needed to produce more viruses.

The new viruses can be made only inside a cell that the virus has infected. The viruses then break open the cell, killing it. Polioviruses do this to nerve cells. As the nerve cells die, muscles no longer work as well. Once it stops working completely, the muscle is paralyzed.

Muscle Fatigue

Treatments with hot packs and exercise may help regain some of the muscle's use. All muscles get tired or fatigued at some point. But a muscle affected by polio will become fatigued more quickly. Here is a simple way to find out when a muscle becomes fatigued.

Hold a hollow rubber ball in the hand you use to write. Keep squeezing the ball as quickly as you can. Have someone keep track of the time and tell you each time fifteen seconds have passed. Count the number of times you squeeze the ball in fifteen seconds. Continue squeezing the ball for three minutes. Have the person write down how many times you squeeze the ball in each fifteen-second period. Your hand muscles become fatigued when the number of times you squeeze the ball starts to drop sharply. Test family members and friends to see when their muscles become fatigued.

As a post-polio syndrome victim, Lauro Halstead today finds that his muscles fatigue easily. Like Salk, Halstead went to medical school. Some forty years after he first got polio, his legs again started to feel weak. At one time, he could jog up six flights of stairs for exercise. But as his leg muscles became weaker, Halstead had to use a motorized scooter to get around. Like Salk, Halstead not only survived but also succeeded. He became director of the post-polio program at the National Rehabilitation Hospital in Washington, D.C.

Chronology

1914—October 28: Jonas is born to Daniel and Dora Salk in New York City.

1916—Polio epidemic strikes New York City, killing more than 2,500 people.

1918—Influenza epidemic strikes America, killing more than 500,000 people.

1926—Jonas attends Townsend Harris High School, where he is interested in history and poetry.

1929—Jonas enters City College of New York at the age of fourteen.

1932—Franklin Delano Roosevelt is elected president.

1934—Salk enters New York University School of Medicine at the age of nineteen. Birthday Balls are held in Roosevelt's honor to raise money for polio research.

1937—The National Foundation for Infantile Paralysis is established.

1938—March of Dimes makes its first appeal for polio research and raises $1.8 million. Salk spends part of his final year in medical school working with Dr. Thomas Francis.

1939—Salk graduates from medical school and marries Donna Lindsay. He starts working as an intern at Mount Sinai Hospital in New York City.

1942—Salk moves to the University of Michigan with his wife and works with Francis on a successful influenza vaccine.

1944—Peter Salk is born.

1947—Darrell Salk is born. Jonas Salk moves to the University of Pittsburgh Medical School where he is given his own lab. He begins work on typing the polioviruses.

1950—Jonathan Salk is born. Jonas Salk begins work on a polio vaccine using killed viruses.

1952—Salk begins testing his vaccine on children at the D. T. Watson Home near Pittsburgh.

1953—Salk announces the results of his vaccine test.

1954—More than 1.8 million children are involved in a national test of the Salk vaccine.

1955—Francis announces that the Salk vaccine is effective. Salk is proclaimed a national hero and is invited to meet with President Dwight D. Eisenhower.

1956—Salk receives the Albert Lasker Award for his work on polio. For the most part, he will be snubbed by his fellow scientists, who do not invite him to join the National Academy of Sciences.

1962—Sabin's live-virus vaccine is introduced in the United States.

1963—The Salk Institute for Biological Studies opens in California.

1968—The Salks get divorced.

1970—Salk marries Françoise Gilot in Paris.

1972—Salk publishes the first of four books on how science affects humankind.

1983—Salk begins research work on AIDS.

1990—Humans are injected in an initial test of an AIDS vaccine prepared by Salk. Results provide information that leads Salk to consider alternative uses of vaccines in AIDS.

1992—Salk announces that he will use his AIDS vaccine therapeutically (post-exposure) rather than preventively (pre-exposure).

1995—June 23: Salk dies from heart failure at the age of eighty.

Chapter Notes

Chapter 1: Innocent Victims

1. Nina Gilden Seavey, Jane S. Smith, and Paul Wagner, *A Paralyzing Fear: The Triumph over Polio in America* (New York: TV Books, 1998), p. 113.

2. "Poliomyelitis—United States, 1940–1995," n.d., <http://nurseweb.ucsf.edu/nip/cdc/polio/polio.html> (August 24, 2001).

3. Peg Kehret, *Small Steps: The Year I Got Polio* (Morton Grove, Ill.: Albert Whitman & Company, 1996), p. 15.

4. Ibid., p. 51.

5. Ibid., p. 53.

6. "A Polio Timeline," *The Polio History Pages*, November 21, 2001, <http://www.cloudnet.com/~edrbsass/poliotimeline.htm> (January 24, 2002).

7. Kehret, p. 169.

Chapter 2: Survival and Success

1. Nina Gilden Seavey, Jane S. Smith, and Paul Wagner, *A Paralyzing Fear: The Triumph over Polio in America* (New York: TV Books, 1998), p. 23.

2. Richard Carter, *Breakthrough: The Saga of Jonas Salk* (New York: Trident Press, 1965), p. 29.

3. "Interview with Jonas Salk, May 16, 1991," *The Hall of Science & Exploration*, May 16, 1991, <http://www.achievement.org/autodoc/page/sal0int-1> (January 24, 2002).

4. Ibid.

5. Ibid.

6. "Influenza 1918," *The American Experience*, n.d., <http://www.pbs.org/wgbh/amex/influenza/filmmore/index.html> (January 24, 2002).

Chapter 3: A Change of Plans

1. "Interview with Jonas Salk, May 16, 1991," *The Hall of Science & Exploration*, May 16, 1991, <http://www.achievement.org/autodoc/page/sal0int-1> (January 24, 2002).

2. Ibid.

3. "Dr. Jonas Salk," n.d., <http://miavx1.muohio.edu/~shermalw/threkeld_salk3.htmlx> (August 24, 2001).

Chapter 4: Relationships

1. "Dr. Jonas Salk," n.d., <http://miavx1.muohio.edu/~shermalw/threkeld_salk3.htmlx> (August 24, 2001)

2. Richard Carter, *Breakthrough: The Saga of Jonas Salk* (New York: Trident Press, 1965), p. 45.

3. Ibid., p. 49.

4. "Interview with Jonas Salk, May 16, 1991," *The Hall of Science & Exploration*, May 16, 1991, <http://www.achievement.org/autodoc/page/sal0int-1> (January 24, 2002).

Chapter 5: His Own Project

1. Dr. Richard Goldbloom, "Family Ties," *Canadian Medical Association Journal*, May 5, 1998, <http://www.cma.ca/cmaj/vol-158/issue-9/1167.htm> (January 24, 2002).

2. Carol Saunders, R.N., "The Vulnerable Among Us: Protection of Children in Medical Research," *Research Practitioner*, March/April 1996, <http://www.researchpractice.com/archive/vuln.shtml> (January 24, 2002)

3. Jane S. Smith, *Patenting the Sun: Polio and the Salk Vaccine* (New York: William Morrow and Company, 1990), p.72.

4. Nina Gilden Seavey, Jane S. Smith, and Paul Wagner, *A Paralyzing Fear: The Triumph over Polio in America* (New York: TV Books, 1998), p. 181.

Chapter 6: His Next Project

1. Nina Gilden Seavey, Jane S. Smith, and Paul Wagner, *A Paralyzing Fear: The Triumph over Polio in America* (New York: TV Books, 1998), p. 195.

2. "Poliomyelitis—United States, 1940–1995," n.d., <http://nurseweb.ucsf.edu/nip/cdc/polio/polio.html> (August 24, 2001).

3. Seavey, p. 181.

Chapter 7: The Polio Vaccine

1. Richard Carter, *Breakthrough: The Saga of Jonas Salk* (New York: Trident Press, 1965), p. 139.

2. Nina Gilden Seavey, Jane S. Smith, and Paul Wagner, *A Paralyzing Fear: The Triumph over Polio in America* (New York: TV Books, 1998), p. 202.

3. Carter, p. 156.

4. Ibid., p. 162.

Chapter 8: The Polio Pioneers

1. George Johnson, "Once Again a Man with a Mission," *New York Times Magazine*, November 25, 1990. p. 60.

2. Richard Carter, *Breakthrough: The Saga of Jonas Salk* (New York: Trident Press, 1965), pp. 214–215.

3. Carter, p. 215.

4. Jane S. Smith, *Patenting the Sun: Polio and the Salk Vaccine* (New York: William Morrow and Company, 1990), p. 318.

5. Carter, p. 316.

6. Ibid., p. 347.

7. Author interview with Dr. Darrell Salk, May 20, 2002.

8. Johnson, p. 60.

9. Nina Gilden Seavey, Jane S. Smith, and Paul Wagner, *A Paralyzing Fear: The Triumph over Polio in America* (New York: TV Books, 1998), pp. 216–217.

Chapter 9: An American Hero

1. Richard Carter, *Breakthrough: The Saga of Jonas Salk* (New York: Trident Press, 1965), p. 264.

2. Jane S. Smith, *Patenting the Sun: Polio and the Salk Vaccine* (New York: William Morrow and Company, 1990), p. 329.

3. Carter, p. 295.

4. Ibid., p. 351.

5. Ibid., p. 354.

6. Ibid., p. 407.

7. *Global Statistical Information & Tables 2001*, July 26, 2002 <http://www.avert.org/globalstats.htm> (September 9, 2002).

8. Charles L. Mee Jr., "The Summer Before Salk," *Esquire*, December 1983, p. 44.

9. "Interview with Jonas Salk, May 16, 1991," *The Hall of Science & Exploration*, May 16, 1991, <http://www.achievement.org/autodoc/page/sal0int-1> (January 24, 2002).

Activities

1. "A Polio Timeline," *The Polio History Pages*, November 21, 2001, <http://www.cloudnet.com/~edrbsass/poliotimeline.htm> (January 24, 2002).

2. Lauro S. Halstead, "Post-Polio Syndrome," *Scientific American*, April 1998, pp. 36–41.

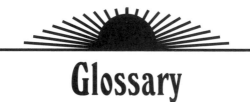

Glossary

Acquired Immune Deficiency Syndrome (AIDS)—Disease caused by a virus that destroys the immune system.

antibody—Chemical made by the body when infected by a virus or bacteria.

attenuated virus—Virus weakened by growing it in an unnatural environment.

bacteria—Tiny living things, also known as microbes, that can cause a variety of diseases.

bacteriology—Study of bacteria.

biochemistry—Study of the chemicals in living things.

control group—Those in a study or experiment who get a placebo.

diaphragm—Muscle that controls breathing.

double-blind test—Test where neither the subjects in the study nor the people responsible for the study know who is getting what.

epidemic—Spread of a disease over a large area so that many people are infected.

experimental group—Those in a study or experiment who get the treatment.

germ—Common name for bacteria or viruses that cause disease.

human immunodeficiency virus (HIV)—The virus that causes AIDS.

immune system—Body's main defense against diseases.

immunity—Protection against a particular disease, like polio.

infantile paralysis—Term for polio.

iron lung—Machine that does the breathing for a person paralyzed by polio.

nucleic acid—Chemical that carries information in all living things and also in viruses.

placebo—Harmless substance given to a person in an experiment.

polio—Disease caused by a virus that can result in paralysis or even death.

poliomyelitis—Full, scientific name for polio.

post-polio syndrome—Symptoms that appear many years after a poliovirus infection.

protein—Chemical that makes up the outer layer of a virus.

tissue culture—Method for growing something, such as a virus, in laboratory glassware.

toxin—Poison produced by bacteria.

vaccination—Injecting a person to prevent a disease.

virus—Particle that can infect cells to cause disease.

white blood cell—Cell that helps fight infection.

Further Reading

Bankston, John. *Jonas Salk and the Polio Vaccine.* Bear, Del.: Mitchell Lane Publishers, Inc., 2001.

Gould, Tony. *A Summer Plague: Polio and Its Survivors.* New Haven, Conn.: Yale University Press, 1997.

McPherson, Stephanie Sammartino. *Jonas Salk: Conquering Polio.* Minneapolis, Minn.: The Lerner Publishing Group, 2001.

Seavey, Nina Gilden, Jane S. Smith, and Paul Wagner. *A Paralyzing Fear: The Triumph Over Polio in America.* New York: TV Books, 1998.

Sherrow, Victoria. *Polio Epidemic: Crippling Virus Outbreak.* Berkeley Heights, N.J.: Enslow Publishers, Inc., 2001.

Internet Addresses

The Jonas Salk Trust
http://www.Jonas-Salk.org/

The Salk Institute for Biological Studies
http://www.salk.edu/

The March of Dimes
http://www.modimes.org/

Jonas Salk, M.D.: Developer of Polio Vaccine
http://www.achievement.org/autodoc/page/sal0bio-1

Index

poliovirus research, 50,
   55–58, 60–69
publications of, 77–78, 104
radio speech, 79
young childhood of,
   19–23, 25
Salk Institute for Biological
   Studies, 101
Salk, Jonathan (son), 76
Salk, Peter (son), 43
Schuulze, Peg, 10, 17–18
See It Now, 95
smallpox, 31, 32, 33

T
tetanus, 32
tissue cultures, 58, 61, 65
Townsend Harris High
   School, 23
toxins, 32–33
Troan, John, 58–59

U
University of Michigan, 43,
   45
University of Pittsburgh
   School of Medicine, 46,
   87

V
vaccination process, 32–35,
   44
viruses, 14, 15–17, 30, 38,
   105, 112–113

W
Watson Home, 71, 74
Weaver, Harry, 47
white blood cells, 33, 61–62
World War II, 42

Y
yellow fever, 33